2023 DEMI OVERVIEW
(Update of Dementia Types, Symptoms, & Risk Factors)

JERRY BELLER HEALTH RESEARCH

Copyright © 2022 Jerry Beller
All rights reserved.
ISBN-13: 9781658764407

DEDICATION

To people living with dementia and their loved ones.

CONTENTS

FOREWORD 1

I. LEWY BODY (LBD) 6

Chapter 1: LEWY BODY DEMENTIA 7

Chapter 2: WHAT IS LEWY BODY DEMENTIA (LBD)? 13

Chapter 3: A-SYNUCLEIN 14

Chapter 4: DEMENTIA WITH LEWY BODIES (DLB)? 17

Chapter 5: DEMENTIA WITH LEWY BODIES (DLB) SYMPTOMS 21

Chapter 6: PARKINSON'S DISEASE (PD)? 24

Chapter 7: PARKINSON'S DISEASE DEMENTIA (PDD) SYMPTOMS 29

II. FTD-RELATED DEMENTIAS 32

Chapter 8: WHAT IS FRONTOTEMPORAL DEMENTIA? 33

Chapter 9: bvFTD BEHAVIORAL VARIANT FRONTOTEMPORAL DEMENTIA? 38

Chapter 10: WHAT IS PROGRESSIVE SUPRANUCLEAR PALSY (PSP)? 43

PSP Life Expectancy 44

III. PRIMARY PROGRESSIVE APHASIA 48

Chapter 11: WHAT IS PRIMARY PROGRESSIVE APHASIA (PPA)? 49

Chapter 12: NONFLUENT/AGRAMMATICAL VARIANT OF PRIMARY PROGRESSIVE APHASIA (naPPA) 54

Chapter 13: LOGOPENIC PROGRESSIVE APHASIA (LPA) 56

Chapter 14: SEMANTIC PRIMARY PROGRESSIVE APHASIA (sPPA) 58

IV. VASCULAR RELATED DEMENTIAS 61

Chapter 15: WHAT IS VASCULAR-DEMENTIA? 62

Chapter 16: CORTICAL VASCULAR DEMENTIA 65

Chapter 17: SUBCORTICAL DEMENTIA/BINSWANGER DISEASE 68

V. ALZHEIMER'S-RELATED DEMENTIAS 70

Chapter 18: WHAT IS ALZHEIMER'S DISEASE? 71

HOW MUCH DOES ALZHEIMER'S COST? 82

Chapter 19: EARLY-ONSET ALZHEIMER'S DISEASE (EOAD) 88

Chapter 20: LIMBIC-PREDOMINANT AGE-RELATED TDP-43 (LATE) OR MEDIAL TEMPORAL ATROPHY 101

Chapter 21: POSTERIOR CORTICAL ATROPHY 108

VI. OTHER DEMENTIAS 111

Chapter 22: AMYOTROPHIC LATERAL SCLEROSIS 112

Chapter 23: CHRONIC TRAUMATIC ENCEPHALOPATHY (CTE) 118

Chapter 24: CORTICOBASAL SYNDROME (CBS) 123

Chapter 25: CREUTZFELDT-JAKOB DISEASE 127

Chapter 26: HUNTINGTON'S DISEASE (HD) 133

Chapter 27: HYDROCEPHALUS 139

Chapter 28: WERNICKE-KORSAKOFF SYNDROME 147

VIII. UPDATES 153

Chapter 29: HAVE WE BEEN BARKING UP THE WRONG TREE WITH BETA-AMYLOID PLAQUES THEORY? 154

Chapter 30: DEMENTIA TESTING 157

CONCLUSION 161

ABOUT THE AUTHOR 170

ACKNOWLEDGMENTS

Thanks to the American Academy of Neurology, Atlanta Center for Medical Research, Alzheimer's Association, Alzheimer's Disease Center, Alzheimer's Disease Center of Northwestern University, Alzheimer's Foundation of America, American Academy of Neurology, Association for Frontotemporal Degeneration, Australia Neurological Research, CDC, Department of Health and Human Services, Duke University Medical Center, Emory Hospital, Harvard Medical School, Johns Hopkins Medicine, Mayo Clinic, National Aphasia Association, National Institute of Neurological Disorders and Strokes, National Library of Medicine, National Institute on Aging, National Institutes of Health, Prince of Wales Medical Research Institute, *PubMed*, Stanford Library School of Medicine, Stanford Medicine, UCSF Department of Neurology, UCSF Memory and Aging Center, University of Cambridge Neurology Unit, World Health Organization (WHO), *Journal of American Medical Association* (JAMA), and several other organizations that provided information used for this book. Thanks to everybody who assisted this book in a variety of important ways, and everybody at Beller Health Research Institute. To my editor, John Briggs, who helps me improve every book. To all sources and for the photos. Most of all, thanks to my wife, Nicola Beller.

2022 DEMENTIA OVERVIEW (Update of Dementia Types, Symptoms, & Risk Factors)

FOREWORD

According to the Saga Populous Poll[1], people fear Alzheimer's and other dementias far more than cancer, heart disease, diabetes, and depression combined. With no cure for most dementia and the severity of these neurological diseases, people understandably feel hopeless. Losing memories and what makes us are perhaps the scariest part of life for anybody who goes through the ordeal.

I am the first to write books on all 19 dementias and one of the thousands of neurologists, researchers, or writers engaged full time in the dementia war. The audience is medical professionals, dementia families and caregivers, and anybody who wants a quick dementia overview.

This book is vital because 4 in 5 Americans are unfamiliar with mild cognitive impairment (MCI), even though 12% to 18% of people older than sixty live with MCI, and over a third of MCI patients develop Alzheimer's[2]. Yet, most Americans confuse MCI with normal aging[3]. Ninety percent of primary care physicians report difficulty determining when MCI ends and Alzheimer's begins.

Patients are not the only ones perplexed by MCI. Over a third of primary care physicians lack confidence in diagnosing MCI, and over half admit confusion about diagnosing MCI because of the similarity to other Alzheimer's symptoms[4].

As you can see, the confusion is monumental, even when we restrict the conversation to MCI and Alzheimer's. The problem is Alzheimer's is only one of 19 primary paths to dementia and one of over one hundred total.

I write this book because patients and physicians struggle to distinguish MCI from Alzheimer's. The confusion only thickens when we add Lewy body dementia, vascular dementia, frontotemporal dementia, and the other primary dementia pathways.

Reading this book will not make you an expert on each dementia. Still, you will better distinguish the 19 primary dementia types than the overwhelming majority of people within and without the medical profession.

While each person must determine what type of book you want, I wrote this book for everybody except dementia patients.

Dementia Patients

I do not recommend the book for dementia patients. If physicians recently diagnosed you with dementia, you are the reason I wrote this book. I help you by helping medical professionals, your loved ones, and caregivers better understand the 19 dementias. While most dementia patients can comprehend the material, I wrote the book to educate those who might help you. Therefore, I write directly to neurologists, general practitioners, geriatricians, other medical professionals, professional and volunteer caregivers, and others who want a better understanding of the 19 primary dementias.

Some recently diagnosed patients read the book, and a few send positive emails, but the subject is too heavy for most. Instead, ask a family member or loved one to read this book for you. I am working on a dementia book to help patients respond to a dementia diagnosis.

Medical Professionals

Although better than ever, most medical professionals cannot distinguish between primary dementia types. Even the most outstanding neurologists struggle at times to make the correct diagnosis.

Diagnosing dementia faces two mountains. The first mountain is extensive and includes all dementia research from the earliest medical journals. However, the second mountain is massive, dwarfing the mountain of dementia knowledge. The peak of the unknown still lurks over the medical profession, evading the most gifted neurological researchers who chip away, much like a few hundred people with shovels attempting to dig through Mount Everest. I respect the overwhelming number of neurological researchers and neurologists with an endless fascination for the human brain.

The book provides a general overview of the 19 dementias for practitioners, geriatricians, neuropsychologists, neurologists, medical students, and other medical professionals.

In reducing misdiagnoses, better dementia education among medical professionals ranks behind blood or urine testing for each dementia type. As a physician, circumstances stack the dementia deck against you like the patient. Diagnosing dementia requires understanding all 19 classes, not just Alzheimer's or a couple. While you need to keep probing each dementia, this book introduces each of the nineteen types on an intermediate level that will benefit most medical professionals.

Dementia Families & Loved Ones

In everyday language, the book helps dementia families and loved ones understand what dementia is, Alzheimer's relationship to dementia, and otherwise distinguish the dementias.

The book does not lend emotional support to dementia families but provides a quick course on the 19 dementias that might help you better understand and deal with your situation.

Which dementia one has often remains undetectable for years, or perhaps until a postmortem autopsy. By understanding the different dementias and the complexities in diagnosing each, you can better appreciate how drawn out and necessary the average dementia diagnosis is. Up to half or more dementia patients develop more than one dementia type, so this book teaches you how to better prepare for that probability.

You will know how important it is for your loved one to see a neurologist or geriatrician trained in all 19 primary dementia diagnoses. The best primary care physician in the world did not learn enough to distinguish between dementias in medical school and probably not in practice. Dementia misdiagnoses are too frequent, and the consequences are often devastating. Medications that ease one dementia's symptoms make them worse for another.

We are introducing a new series for dementia families and loved ones, which will address you directly, but this book addresses a broad audience, including you.

Caregivers

The book offers caregivers a relatively quick overview of the most prevalent dementia types. Most professional caregivers who care for dozens of dementia patients know more about dementia than the average primary care physician (not criticizing physicians).

Whether a professional or a voluntary caregiver, this book helps caregivers understand the different dementias and what to expect with the dementia process. You still must read other books on caregiving, but this book helps you better understand the terrible forms of dementia inflicting people under your care.

Let's discuss what this book is and is not.

What this book is

- The book is an intermediate discussion of dementia
- Where possible, we use common everyday language
- We meticulously cite references to hundreds of studies and other authorities
- The first book to summarize all 19 dementias causing 99% of dementia
- We describe each dementia type
- We list and briefly discuss each associated symptom
- We discuss causes, if known, for each dementia
- We discuss prevalence for the United States, globally, and for other countries in various sections of the book

What this book is not

- While we touch on caregiving, this is not a book on caregiving
- We discuss steps dementia families should take, but this is not the book's primary purpose
- This book has a diagnosis value, but is not a diagnosis book
- The book covers all 19 dementia types on an intermediate micro level. The companion book in the series, *Dementia Overview: The Umbrella View*, takes a macro view, covering the dementia umbrella

Dementia types

When the dementia discussion expands beyond Alzheimer's disease, the topic usually becomes one of Alzheimer's, Lewy body dementia, vascular dementia, and perhaps frontotemporal dementia.

However, there are not one but several forms of Alzheimer's, Lewy body dementia, vascular dementia, and frontotemporal dementia. Depending on the pathology and associated protein, others fall into the category *other dementias*.

Alzheimer's Disease

- Typical Alzheimer's
- Early-onset Alzheimer's
- Limbic-predominant age-related TDP-43 (LATE)
- Posterior cortical atrophy

Lewy Body Dementia

- Dementia with Lewy bodies
- Parkinson's disease dementia

Vascular Dementia

- Cortical (post-stroke & multi-infarct) vascular dementia
- Subcortical (Binswanger disease) vascular dementia

Frontotemporal Dementia

- Behavioral variant frontotemporal dementia (bvFTD)
- Progressive supranuclear palsy

Primary Progressive Aphasia (PPA)

- Nonfluent-agrammatic variant primary progressive aphasia
- Logopenic Progressive Aphasia
- Semantic primary progressive aphasia

Other Dementias

- Amyotrophic lateral sclerosis
- Chronic traumatic encephalopathy
- Corticobasal syndrome
- Creutzfeldt-Jakob disease
- Huntington's disease
- Hydrocephalus
- Wernicke-Korsakoff syndrome

We added another category for primary progressive aphasias. Although most list them in the frontotemporal dementia category, we give primary progressive aphasias their class because their pathologies include frontotemporal, Alzheimer's, and others.

This book combines the information from all nineteen other books on singular dementias, providing an invaluable quick study for anybody inside or outside the medical profession who wants to understand dementia better.

I write the book in American English but include quotes from around the world and ask Americans to respect the different spellings in the international quotations and people from the UK, Australia, Canada, and elsewhere to accept the book's information within the framework of my American English.

I. LEWY BODY (LBD)

How is it, one fine morning, Duchenne discovered a disease which probably existed in the time of Hippocrates?

— Jean-Martin Charcot

    Charcot is one of my favorite historical figures. His question about medical discoveries reminds me of an Italian captain who commissioned a ship with the Spanish monarchy to find a passageway to India, got lost, and "discovered" an already inhabited continent (New World). Even though he got lost and stumbled upon an inhabited continent, Vikings and perhaps other Europeans also had already "discovered," the people of the continent celebrate the lost one's name as the great discoverer.

    Neither Charcot's quote, nor my spin, undermine the medical contributions of the physicians and researchers in this book credited with advancing our understanding of the various disorders. The quote's point is that more than one person is involved in discovering any medical problem. If the medical problem predates any one person by hundreds or thousands of years, physicians around the globe have been observing and trying to figure out the same medical issue.

    Charcot's question points out the impossibility of building any timeline for most disorders without leaving out dozens who did much of the heavy lifting. I purposely leave out no critical players in developing each dementia type. Observations of most dementias go back to ancient times, well before recorded history. Our goal is to provide a general historical context; with the stipulation, it would be impossible not to leave out key players' historians either failed to record or got lost or destroyed.

Chapter 1: LEWY BODY DEMENTIA

Lewy body dementia is a combination of Parkinson's and cognitive issues associated with other dementia types, such as Alzheimer's.

What is Lewy Body Dementia (LBD)?

Protein buildups are prevalent in most dementias, and Lewy body dementia (LBD) is no different.

"Protein deposits, called Lewy bodies," said the Mayo Clinic, "develop in nerve cells in the brain regions involved in thinking, memory and movement[5] (motor control)."

The Lewy Body Association[6] provides a similar definition.

> *Lewy body dementia (LBD) is a progressive brain disorder in which Lewy bodies (abnormal deposits of a protein called alpha-synuclein) build up in areas of the brain that regulate behavior, cognition, and movement.*

Research links rogue protein to Alzheimer's, vascular dementia, and other dementias. In Lewy body dementia, we focus on alpha synuclein protein.

Is there a cure for Lewy body dementia?

Like most dementias, there is no cure for Lewy body dementia, but early detection remains essential to slow and treat symptoms[7]. Governments and corporations must invest more in independent research to discover tests, vaccines, and treatments for each primary dementia to find a cure.

While no cure exists, we can do much to prevent this and other dementias.

What causes Lewy body dementia?

Science does not know what causes LBD but focuses on a protein buildup, alpha synuclein, that clumps into Lewy bodies.

Alpha-synuclein

Experts long ago linked rogue protein to dementia. Researchers from the University of California San Francisco Medical Center confirmed alpha synuclein is a double-edged sword.

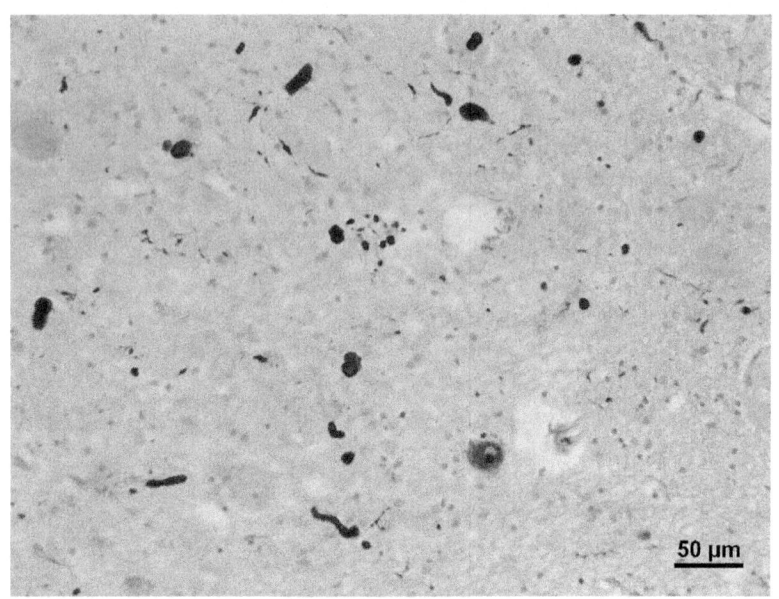

Lewy bodies (alpha synuclein inclusions) [8]

The study's lead author Robert Edwards, MD, discussed the results. High levels of Lewy bodies (alpha synuclein) present in Parkinson's disease inhibit fusion between vesicles and membranes, "necessary for neurotransmitter release," said Edwards. "But in normal amounts, it has a {different} effect: if neurotransmitters are already being released, alpha-synuclein helps speed the process[9]."

Scientists must learn if the protein forms to protect the neurons or if mutated genes destroy the neuron network related to many motor and non-motor skills.

Lewy Bodies

Lewy bodies result when alpha synuclein protein develops clumps and deposits. Alpha synuclein forms in the brain stem and clumps cause "resting tremor," slowness, and stiffness.

The protein clumps kill neurons and attack the brain's elaborate communication system, causing Lewy body dementia symptoms.

The deposits can also affect the cortex area of the brain and inhibit cognitive skills. We soon discuss the symptoms the deposits produce.

Cortex

The cortex is the outside layer of the brain inhabited by millions of neurons[10]. When many think of the brain, they form an image of the cortex.

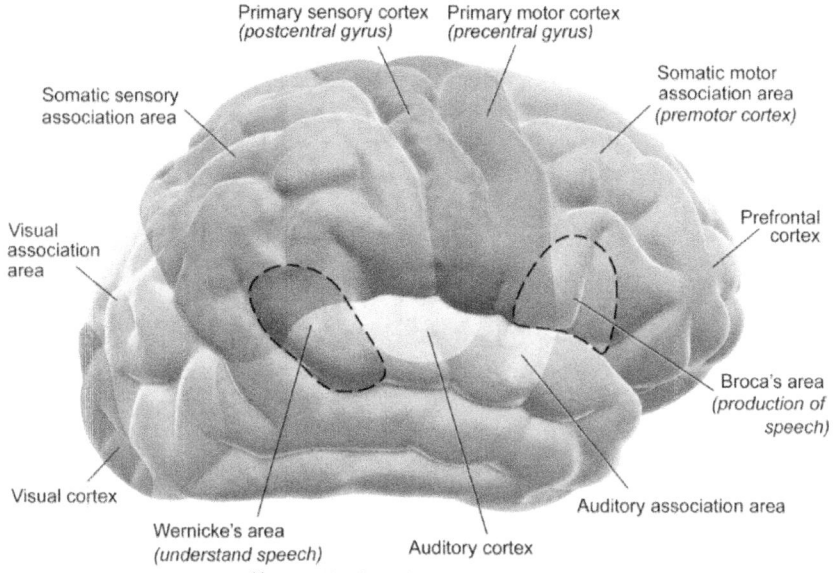

Source[11]: Medical gallery of Blausen Medical 2014

The brain depends on the cortex for sensory skills. Let's discuss the seven cortex areas.

7 Cortex Areas

1. Primary visual cortex is in the occipital lobe[12]
2. Primary auditory cortex above the temporal lobe[13]
3. Primary somatosensory cortex is behind the central sulcus[14]
4. Secondary somatosensory cortex by the lateral fissure[15]
5. Primary motor cortex sits in front of the primary somatosensory cortex[16]
6. Premotor cortex resides in the section of the motor cortex in the frontal lobe[17]
7. Pre-frontal cortex locates in front of the pre-motor cortex[18]

The different layers of the cortex and the neurons within manage our movement and cognitive skills. When the protein deposits damage the neurons, our sensory and motor skills break down.

Two Lewy Body Dementia (LBD) Types

There are two versions of Lewy body dementia:
1. Dementia with Lewy bodies (DLB)
2. Parkinson's disease dementia (PDD)

Dementia with Lewy bodies and PDD pose opposite routes to the same neurological disorder.

The University of California, San Francisco, provides an informative overview:

> *Lewy body dementias include dementia with Lewy bodies (DLB) and Parkinson's disease with dementia (PDD) and are the second most frequent cause of dementia in elderly adults. These degenerative brain diseases {are associated} with abnormal clumps of a protein called alpha-synuclein. These clumps, called Lewy bodies, {are} in nerve cells throughout the outer layer of the brain (the cerebral cortex) and deep inside the midbrain and brainstem. Patients with these diseases experience progressive cognitive decline, although there is considerable variability in symptoms between patients. Common symptoms include problems with movement, visual hallucinations, and fluctuations in thinking skills or attention*[19].

According to John Hopkins Health Library[20], over 1.4 million Americans suffer from one of the two forms of Lewy body dementia[21].

Misdiagnosis

Lewy Body Dementia Association (LBDA) warns that many doctors are unaware or don't understand Lewy body dementia and misdiagnose many patients who go untreated, under-treated, or maltreated.

Compared to past generations, there's much more information today a primary care physician must learn. I also stress again there is no accurate blood or urine test for dementia as there is for cancer and other diseases (Hello Congress!).

Note to Doctors & Medical Professionals

When treating Parkinson's-like symptoms, doctors should resist the urge to prescribe antipsychotic drugs. According to LBDA, such drugs cause neuroleptic malignant syndrome in people who have dementia with Lewy bodies or Parkinson-related dementia[22].

The combination of misdiagnosis and the resulting antipsychotic medication shut down kidneys and speeds up the most devastating effects of dementia, including death.

Note to public

Choosing the right doctor is more important than ever. Being medical-book-smart is insufficient to diagnose and treat dementia because medical books remain incomplete.

To diagnose dementia, one must never stop learning and do their best to keep up and make sense of the ongoing critical medical studies on all diseases doctors treat.

Dementia overwhelms the primary care physician and challenges the best neurologists. You must be the first care provider for your health, helping the doctor and medical officials by documenting your symptoms, making a doctor's appointment as soon as neurological symptoms develop, and helping them fill in the pieces of the puzzle.

Patients trust doctors to make most dementia-related decisions with an incomplete handbook. Besides diagnosing and treating hundreds of other potential medical issues their patients face, doctors must tread through mountains and valleys of conflicting dementia information.

Without accurate urine or blood tests for most dementias, we demand the impossible from primary care physicians.

Misdiagnosis is not simply a matter of having or not having money or having good insurance—although those are factors. Diagnosing dementia is a guessing game, guaranteeing widespread misdiagnosis.

When Robin Williams died, news outlets reported depression drove him to suicide. However, his autopsy showed Williams suffered Lewy body dementia, which had gone undiagnosed.

Doctors diagnosed and treated Robin Williams for Parkinson's disease. Still, only the autopsy confirmed the Lewy bodies had spread through his brain, evidence to Lewy body dementia, or in his case, Parkinson's disease dementia (PDD). After the autopsy, specialists debate whether Williams had dementia with Lewy bodies or Parkinson's disease dementia. Dennis Dickson, MD, Mayo Clinic, and an LBDA Scientific Advisory Council member analyzed the coroner's report.

"Mr. Williams {received} a clinical diagnosis of PD and [was] treated for motor symptoms," said Dr. Dickson. "The report confirms he experienced depression, anxiety, and paranoia, which may occur in either Parkinson's disease or dementia with Lewy bodies."

I complain again we do not have a simple, accurate test or cure for Parkinson's disease, Parkinson's disease dementia, dementia with Lewy bodies, Alzheimer's disease, and most dementias.

The world's governments should be ashamed for not supporting and funding the research for scientists to conduct the studies to develop an accurate and cheap test and cure for these devastating diseases. Indeed, dozens of smaller studies show promising results but need funding for more extensive studies to confirm and make available to the public.

What Is The Difference Between Dementia With Lewy Bodies (DLB) And Parkinson's Disease Dementia (PDD)?

Dementia with Lewy bodies (DLB) and Parkinson's disease dementia (PDD) are two paths to Lewy body Dementia (LBD).

A *Fifth Department of Internal Medicine* study explains it is difficult to distinguish between DLB and PDD, except dementia strikes before Parkinsonism in the former, whereas Parkinsonism predates dementia in the latter. Otherwise, "there are few or no pathological differences between DLB and PDD," according to the Fukuoka University study[23].

Ester Heerema, MSW, and Claudia Chaves, MD, explain why it is difficult to distinguish between dementia with Lewy bodies and Parkinson's disease with dementia. "Symptoms that affect the body include muscle weakness, rigidity (stiffness), and slowness in movements," said Heerema. "Symptoms in the brain include impaired executive functioning, attention span, and memory loss."

Patients with DLB and PDD suffer from depression and hallucinations.

Are PDD and DLB different versions of the same disease?

DLB and PDD are the same neurological disorders but have different origins, sharing many symptoms, but the occurrence varies. Physicians must perform a cognitive assessment to distinguish between DLB and PDD.

Cognitive decline is systematic in PDD and DLB but develops differently. DLB causes varying levels of cognitive ability, whereas PDD produces a steadier cognitive decline. Thus, the cognitive ability of DLB patients shows a drastic improvement in one test, only to decline the next.

DLB begins as dementia and develops Parkinson's disease, while Parkinson's with Lewy bodies begins as Parkinson's disease before developing dementia.

Physicians base their hypothesis on how patients answer questions to determine if somebody is suffering from PDD or DLB. The patient and family should document the symptoms in a medical journal and complete a report. You never know when such a medical journal might save your life or prolong the quality. Provide your doctor with full access.

And express the whole truth when the doctor asks questions. Once a neurologist or other physician understands the symptoms, they should conduct a cognitive assessment.

How else do medical experts distinguish between PDD and DLB?

Once the diseases advance, PDD and DLB are the same from a clinical standpoint. If dementia precedes Parkinson's disease, it is DLB. Thus, dementia as an early symptom is the primary difference between PDD and DLB.

Experts admit the peculiar distinction, two paths to the same combination of Parkinson's disease and Lewy body dementia. However, if we've learned anything from dementia research, there are many more types or subtypes than we ever imagine.

Chapter 2: WHAT IS LEWY BODY DEMENTIA (LBD)?

People make some of the most significant discoveries in their late teens and early twenties. When 26, Albert Einstein released (then) groundbreaking scientific papers on Brownian motion[24], special relativity[25], photoelectric effect[26], and the equivalence of mass and energy[27].

When his doctor-father complained about the limitations of the echocardiogram, 15-year-old Suman Mulumudi[28] used a 3-D printer to develop the Steth IO, which provides better sound than the stethoscope and comes with a visual graph. At 22, Galileo published a book outlining his design of hydrostatic balance[29]. At age 16, in 1642, Blaise Pascal[30] developed the first calculating devices and prototypes, leading to the computer revolution.

A young person also discovered Lewy body dementia.

In 1912, German Dr. Friedrich H. Lewy[31] discovered Lewy body dementia (LBD) while analyzing Parkinson's disease[32].

Although later persecuted as a Jew (he and his wife fled to the United States during W.W. II), Dr. Lewy discovered Lewy body dementia only two years after completing medical school. Dr. Lewy is a testament to what young people can accomplish and how a person can overcome significant hardship.

Despite Dr. Lewy's key role, the Parkinsonism story neither begins nor ends with Lewy or Lewy bodies, as we soon discuss in the Parkinson's disease and dementia with Lewy bodies sections.

Lewy bodies (alpha-synuclein)

In the early twentieth century, older scientists passed the baton to younger scientists who eagerly built on the work of the ancient Indians, Galen, Parkinson, Charcot, and others. A few years after he identified Alzheimer's disease, one of Dr. Alzheimer's assistants, Dr. Fredrich Lewy, just three years out of medical school, discovered Lewy bodies in 1912 while examining a Parkinson's brain during the autopsy.

Lewy body dementia (LBD)

We associate Lewy bodies with Parkinsonism neurological disorders falling under the umbrella term Lewy body dementia (LBD).

1. Dementia with Lewy bodies
2. Parkinson's disease
3. Parkinson's disease dementia

There are other Parkinsonism disorders, but these three are the most prevalent and related. A-synuclein clumps connect the Lewy body dementias.

Chapter 3: A-SYNUCLEIN

Most dementia discussions center on "rogue protein."
Encoded by the SNCA gene, alpha-synuclein (a-synuclein) is in the heart tissue and muscle, but mainly in the presynaptic terminals on the tips of neurons in the central nervous system, in the cerebellum, hippocampus, neocortex, substantia nigra, and thalamus.

Whatever positive roles a-synuclein play in the neural process, it kills neurons when it turns rogue and overproduces. It disrupts the synaptic terminals, resulting in Parkinson's disease, DLB, or another neurological disorder.

The Department of Anatomy and Structural Biology at Albert Einstein College of Medicine[33] investigated a-synuclein relationship with Parkinson's and Lewy body dementia. It concluded a "wild-type alpha-synuclein {selectively translocated} into lysosomes for degradation by the chaperone-mediated autophagy pathway." It acted as uptake blockers, "inhibiting both their own degradation and that of other substrates."

Please view the structural model of human a-synuclein in the image below.

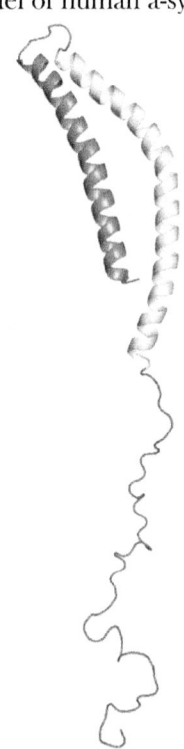

A structural model of human alpha-synuclein[34]

Vital in the formation and stabilization of synapse, a-synuclein is a presynaptic protein comprising 140 amino acids[35]. Flexible, a-synuclein mixes conformational plasticity and adaptability to environmental force. Alpha-synuclein begins natively unfolded, but in response to environmental influences, the protein partially folds or folds into monomers, polymers, oligomers, amorphous aggregates, or fibrils resembling amyloid or some combination[36].

Alpha-synuclein & Neurogeneration

The image illustrates the a-synuclein protein aggregation pathway.

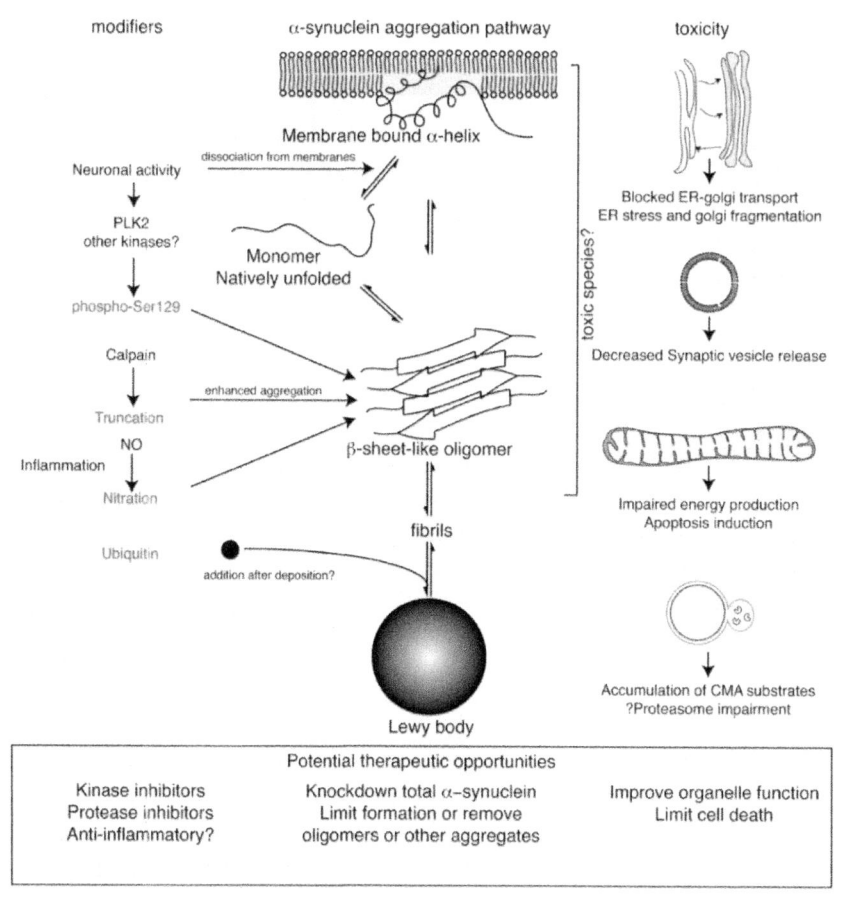

A-synuclein and Neuronal Cell Death[37]

The image left shows a slow brewing toxic storm leading to Lewy body clunks in the middle. Image right follows the consequences, including blocked ERgolgi transport ER stress and fragmentation, synaptic vesicle release impairment, diminished energy production apoptosis induction, and CMA substrates proteasome accumulation[38].

Scientists must learn if the protein forms to protect the neurons or mutated genes destroy the neuron network related to motor and non-motor skills. Several neurologists, including Dale Bredesen and David Perlmutter, argue that overactive proteins are an effect, not the cause. They claim the protein deposits associated with dementias are protective mechanisms in response to underlying causes such as viruses like herpes, oral infections, toxins, and inflammation.

Bredesen's view might explain why all dementia drug trials fail. By focusing on the actual causes, researchers stand a better chance of developing tests, vaccines, and cures for each dementia type.

Synaptic Process

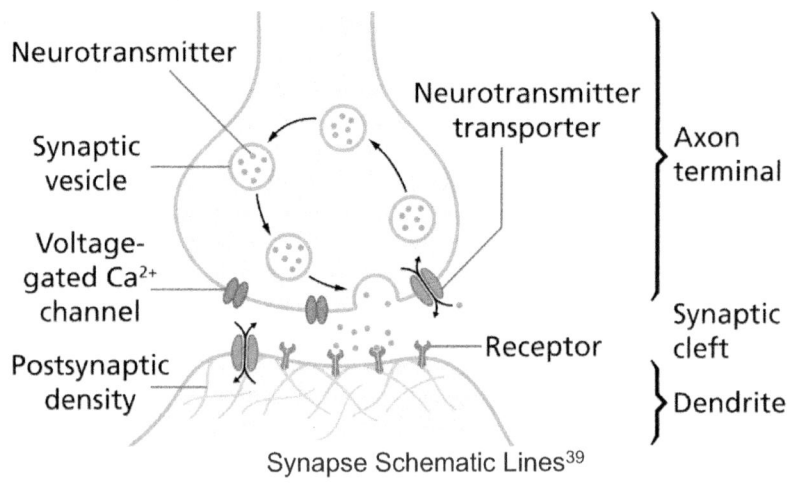

Synapse Schematic Lines[39]

Researchers do not know a-synuclein's exact role as several proteins and cytoskeletal elements relate to synapses' synaptic vesicle release cycle[40]. A-synuclein plays a not fully understood role in lipid rafts[41] and the distal pool of synaptic vesicles[42].

Astbury Center for Structural Biology researchers discovered the C-terminal and N-terminal regions a-synuclein act as master controllers for aggregation and function. Study coauthor Sheena Radford, PhD, director of the Astbury Center for Structural Biology in the UK, explained the importance. "Our discovery of master controller regions may open up new opportunities to understand how mutating the protein sequence that causes disease could help us find the Achilles heel for these proteins to target for future therapeutic intervention[43]."

The study allows future studies to develop the means to control rogue proteins. "Future research can also look at whether other proteins involved in different diseases also have master controller regions of aggregation," said Radford, "which could open up new avenues for therapeutic development in several neurodegenerative diseases which involve the aggregation of disordered proteins like alpha-synuclein."

Now, let's discuss the two Lewy body dementias caused by a-synuclein, dementia with Lewy bodies, and Parkinson's disease dementia.

Chapter 4: DEMENTIA WITH LEWY BODIES (DLB)?

People with DLB have a buildup of abnormal protein particles in their brain tissue, called Lewy bodies. Lewy bodies are {in} the brain tissue of people with Parkinson's disease (PD) and Alzheimer's disease (AD). However, in these conditions, the Lewy bodies are {in} different parts of the brain.

The presence of Lewy bodies in DLB, PD, and AD suggests a connection among these conditions. But scientists haven't yet figured out what the connection is.

DLB affects a person's ability to think, reason, and process information. It can also affect movement, personality, and memory.

–Cedars-Sinal[44]

The connection between dementia with Lewy bodies (DLB) and Parkinson's disease dementia (PDD) is undeniable but not fully understood. Are DLB and PDD the same neurological disorder?

One glaring difference between Parkinson's disease dementia (PDD) and dementia with Lewy bodies (DLB) is Parkinson's begins as Parkinson's disease and no dementia. However, science cannot confirm if they are the same or two different neurological disorders caused by Lewy bodies.

Many publications refer to dementia with Lewy bodies (DLB) and Lewy body dementia (LBD) inter-exchangeably, but they are not synonymous. If Dementia with Lewy bodies and Lewy body dementia is the same, by the same logic, so would be Parkinson's disease dementia. For this book, dementia with Lewy bodies and Parkinson's disease dementia are two branches of the umbrella term Lewy body dementia.

Alzheimer's Association describes dementia with Lewy bodies[45] (DLB) as: "a progressive dementia that leads to a decline in thinking, reasoning, and independent function because of abnormal microscopic deposits that damage brain cells."

Dementia with Lewy bodies (DLB) History

In 1912, Russian Konstantin Tretiakoff[46] named the alpha-synuclein[47] deposits "Lewy body" in honor of Dr. Friedrich Lewy. By 1961, Japanese Okazaki connected cortical Lewy bodies and dementia.

In 1980, Japanese psychiatrist, Kenji Kosaka, recommended the term "Lewy body dementia." Fifteen years later, in 1995, the DLB International Consortium acted on Kosaka's proposal and made Lewy body dementia (LBD) the official umbrella term for the following Parkinsonism disorders:

- Parkinson's disease (PD)
- Parkinson's disease dementia (PDD)
- Dementia with Lewy bodies (DLB)

Neurologists universally accepted Kosaka's recommendations, but many in Japan and a few outside refer to DLB as "Kosaka's disease." His contribution was strong enough to deserve such recognition, but we will use Kosaka's recommended terms, which carry the Lewy name.

The formation of the DLB International Consortium workshop[48] represented a significant step forward for Lewy body dementia research. The consortium set the DLB diagnosis criteria in 1995, revised it in 2003, again in 2009, and in 2017 the last update[49].

Although under political attack during the COVID-19 pandemic, the National Institute on Health and several other health organizations in the US, Newcastle University in the UK, and several international health organizations fund the DLB International Consortium. Those attacking health organizations such as NIH act clueless of their critical role in financing significant medical research.

The consortium sets the bar high for DLB and Lewy body research. They maintain focus among researchers and provide strong leadership. The accumulative work of the ancient Indian physicians Galen, Parkinson, Charcot, Lewy, and Tretiakoff, and others led to the all-star neurological team comprising the DLB International Consortium.

How prevalent is dementia with Lewy bodies?

About 1.4 million Americans[50], a minimum of 100,000 in the UK[51],

and 5-10% of people living with dementia worldwide live with dementia with Lewy bodies[52][53][54] (DLB).

According to many sources[55][56][57][58], besides Alzheimer's, dementia with Lewy bodies (DLB) destroys more lives than any singular dementia.

However, many reduce the dementias to the following categories.

- Alzheimer's disease (AD)
- Lewy body dementia (LBD)
- Vascular dementia
- Frontotemporal dementia (FTD)
- Non-categorized dementias.

When grouped in the more general categories, authorities often list vascular dementia second[59][60][61][62] and Lewy body dementia (DLB and Parkinson's disease dementia) third.

Non-categorized dementias include normal pressure hydrocephalus, Huntington's disease, Korsakoff syndrome, Creutzfeldt-Jakob disease, amyotrophic lateral sclerosis, HIV-related cognitive impairment, and chronic traumatic encephalopathy. When you add these dementias together, they still do not break the top four in prevalence.

According to the Lewy Body Dementia Association (LBDA), Lewy bodies are the second most prevalent dementia form. The LBDA claims dementia with Lewy bodies is the most misdiagnosed and underdiagnosed of all dementias[63]. Too many misdiagnoses remain[64][65][66][67], and the data is not current enough or conclusive. However, when addressing singular dementias, DLB is second, but when grouped, the vascular dementias (post-stroke dementia, multi-stroke dementia, and subcortical dementia) are likely second.

Any way you shake dementia statistics, dementia with Lewy bodies accounts for 5 to 25 percent of dementia occurrence (the wide range of possibilities gives me a headache). The rankings remain dubious since the system estimates rather than provides actual data.

Rather than over-focus on debatable rankings, we need better data and prevention measures since risk factors suggest lifestyle changes might prevent much or most dementia cases.

Who does DLB strike?

DLB & gender

Studies conflict on whether DLB strikes males or females more.

An Italian study[68] (Farina, Baglio, et al., 2009) found both sexes equally at risk.

A Chinese study[69] (Yue, Wang, et al., 2016), a Norwegian study[70] (Rongve, Soennesyn, et al., 2015), and an American study[71] (Goodman, Lochner, et al., 2017) found greater DLB incidence in males than females.

Many consider the above and similar studies the gospel, but we must balance such conclusions. Some studies showed only a slightly greater risk for males than females. And the Italian study we led showed the equal risk to both sexes.

Adding further murk, other studies such as a Swedish study[72] {Fereshtehnejad, Religa, et al., 2013} and a UK study[73] {Price, Farooq, et al., 201} showed greater DLB incidence in females than males.

And in agreement with the Italian study, a second French study[74] (Mouton, Blanc, et al., 2018) found no significant difference in DLB risks between the sexes compared to Alzheimer's or Parkinson's.

(Kurasz, Smith, et al., 2020) perhaps shined some light on the conflicting results. Compared to whites, African Americans and Hispanic DLB patients are most likely to be female[75]. The results suggest white males are more likely to get DLB, while African American and Hispanic females carry higher risks.

We need more studies to determine what white males have in common with African American and Hispanic females, placing them at greater risk. Figuring out the link might point researchers towards what causes DLB. While there might be a slightly greater DLB risk for males, it might only be for white males. And the overall difference, if there is one, is too slight to draw the distinction most dementia websites and books do by insisting on a clear greater risk for males.

DLB & race

During the male and female comparison conversation, we learned African American and Hispanic females, along with white men, are high-risk groups. However, we lack credible data to determine which races are the most significant DLB risk. There is a gap in our knowledge, especially for the second or third most prevalent dementia type, another indictment of record-keeping and access to critical medical data locally and globally.

Researchers do not need personal information but medical histories, treatments, and other data to advance science. Such inadequacies make me worry we are squandering our digital era.

What age does DLB strike?

DLB typically strikes people between the ages of fifty and eighty[76].

Early onset DLB

A minority of cases occur before age fifty, called early onset dementia with Lewy bodies (EODLB). Early onset DLB strikes people as young as teens or pre-teens[77]. One difference between dementia and early onset dementia is most early onset dementia is hereditary, but genetics explains only a low percentage of regular dementia.

Dementia with Lewy bodies (DLB) life expectancy

DLB does not kill as fast as Creutzfeldt-Jakob disease and the fastest dementias. Still, neither does it stretch out as long as Alzheimer's or one of the slower-acting dementias like Alzheimer's disease, where people might live up to twenty years following diagnosis.

The average DLB patient lives for 5-8 years from diagnosis[78,79], although some die within two years, and others live up to two decades[80].

Chapter 5: DEMENTIA WITH LEWY BODIES (DLB) SYMPTOMS

Whereas the other books in the series focus primarily on early symptoms likely present at diagnosis, we take a broader look at symptoms in this overview book.

DLB symptoms in each category resemble some dementias. However, signs distinguish DLB from other dementia types. Distinguishing DLB from Alzheimer's, sporadic attention deficits are a key DLB characteristic. Contrasting DLB from Parkinson's disease is the dementia presence.

Once we've gone through the process for each dementia, we will build comparison tables to provide quick and easy access to compare symptoms. Diagnosing dementia, you begin with dozens of neurological possibilities, including dementias. The comparison table helps narrow the dementia possibilities.

With no blood or urine test for each dementia, diagnosis is—more than anything else—a process of elimination. The other books in the series focus on early symptoms and diagnosis techniques, whereas this book does not go as deep but provides a broader overview.

In this chapter, we divide DLB symptoms into five categories:

1. Behavior and mood
2. Cognitive
3. Mobility
4. Sleep
5. Other symptoms

One early sign of dementia with Lewy bodies is failing to read body language and facial expressions. Measuring one's ability to recognize anger, disgust, fear, happiness, sadness, and surprise, a study (Kojima, Hidaka, et al., 2018) found dementia with Lewy body patients only responded to happy facial expressions.

Kohima and team reported:

> *In patients with Lewy body disease, happiness was {unaffected} by aging, age of onset, duration of the disease, cognitive function, and apathy; however, recognizing the facial expression of fear was difficult. In addition, due to aging, cognitive decline, and apathy, the facial expression recognition ability for sadness and anger decreased. In particular, cognitive decline reduced recognition of all {facial} expressions except for happiness. The test accuracy rates were classified {using} the cluster analysis: 'stable type,' 'mixed type,' and 'reduced type.' In the 'reduced type,' the overall*

facial recognition ability declined except happiness, and in the mixed type, {the} recognition ability of anger particularly declined[81].

Facial recognition decline does not prove dementia with Lewy bodies (DLB) but makes it a strong suspect, especially when associated with other DLB symptoms.

DLB Behavioral and Mood Symptoms

People who have dementia with Lewy bodies experience six primary behavioral and mood symptoms.

- Agitation
- Apathy
- Anxiety
- Delusions
- Depression
- Paranoia

DLB Cognitive Symptoms

DLB cognitive symptoms include cognitive fluctuations and dementia. Expect changes in personality, thinking, and reasoning[82]. DLB patients experience confusion, often occurring off and on[83]. DLB produces delusions[84], hallucinations[85], and memory issues that might fluctuate at different parts of the day[86]. Patients usually appear unmotivated[87].

DLB Motor Symptoms

DLB patients suffer a variety of movement problems. DLB patients move slow, unsteady, unsure[88]. As the disease progresses, it causes Parkinson's symptoms, including balance issues and hunching[89]. DLB sufferers also experience problems judging distance[90].

DLB Movement Problems Symptoms include:

- Balance disorder[91]
- Coordination decline
- Blank facial expressions[92]
- Falling[93]
- Muscle rigidity
- Muscle stiffness
- Shaking while resting
- Shuffled walk
- Stooped posture

- Swallowing problems
- Tremor
- Speaking problems[94]
- Writing becomes smaller

DLB Sleep Symptoms

DLB causes daytime sleepiness, insomnia, REM sleep behavior disorder (RBD), and restless leg syndrome. DLB-associated sleep disorders include violent outbursts during uncomfortable dreams[95].

Other DLB Symptoms

DLB patients also suffer choking[96] and fainting[97], blood pressure and body temperature problems, urinary incontinence, and sexual dysfunction. Other symptoms include chest infections[98], constipation, and a diminished sense of smell.

- A diminished sense of smell
- Blood pressure
- Body temperature
- Chest infections
- Choking
- Constipation
- Fainting
- Sexual dysfunction
- Urinary incontinence

Other DLB Sources: Mayo Clinic[99], National Institute on Aging[100] (NIH), Lewy Body Dementia Association[101], National Health Service[102] (NHS).

Chapter 6: PARKINSON'S DISEASE (PD)?

I study all neurological disorders, but Parkinsonism is personal because one of my favorite aunts developed Parkinson's disease (PD). Having written books on all 19 dementias, I follow each close. If I spend extra time with one neurological disorder branch, it is Lewy body dementia, including Parkinson's disease (PD), Parkinson's disease dementia (PDD), and dementia with Lewy bodies (DLB).

The medical community named Parkinson's disease (PD) after Dr. James Parkinson, the British physician who discovered the condition in 1817 and described it in *An Essay on the Shaking Palsy*.

According to the Parkinson's Foundation, Parkinson's disease is a "neurodegenerative disorder that affects predominately dopamine-producing (dopaminergic) neurons in a specific area of the brain called the substantia nigra[103]."

The substantia nigra plays a vital role in any Parkinson's conversation.

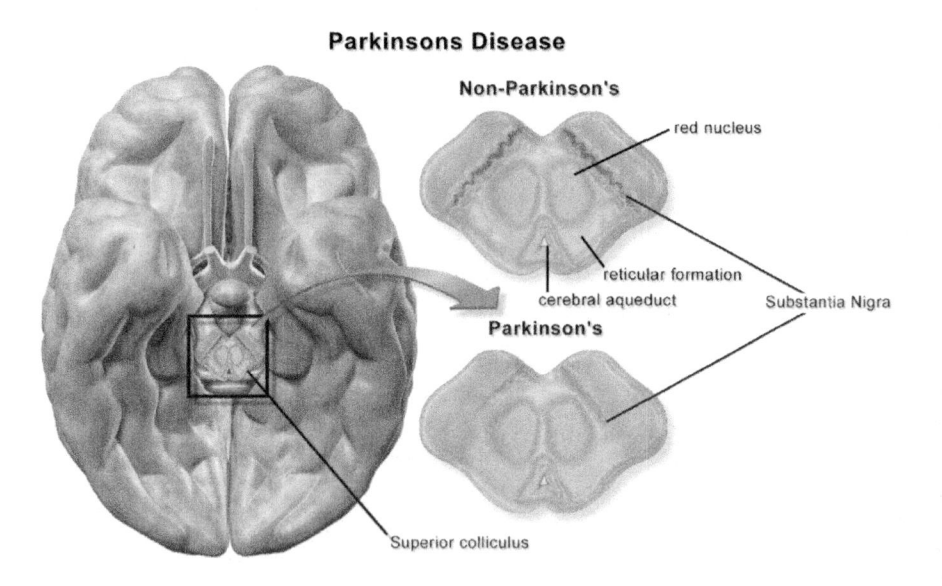

Parkinsons Disease

Non-Parkinson's
red nucleus
reticular formation
cerebral aqueduct
Substantia Nigra
Parkinson's
Superior colliculus

The American Parkinson Disease Association describes Parkinson's disease.

Parkinson's disease is a type of movement disorder that can affect the ability to perform common, daily activities. It is a chronic and progressive disease, meaning that the symptoms become {worse}. It is characterized by its most common of motor symptoms – tremors (rhythmic shaking), stiffness or rigidity of the muscles, and slowness of movement (called bradykinesia) – but also manifests in non-motor symptoms including sleep problems, constipation, anxiety, depression, and fatigue, among others[104].

Before we dive deeper, let's briefly discuss Parkinson's disease (PD) history to see who made some fundamental discoveries. Our historical investigation unraveled a rich past where significant Parkinson's advances coincided with wider medical breakthroughs. Probing Lewy body dementia (LBD), including Parkinson's disease (PD), ingrained an even deeper appreciation for ancient people whose curiosity and devotion to medicine built the foundation that modern medicine sits.

Parkinson's disease (PD) history

Over 3,000 years ago, Indian physicians collaborated orally and then in writing and created the Ayurveda[105] (science of life or life knowledge).

Ayurveda described Parkinsonism in 600 BC *Sushruta Samhita*[106] medical and surgical text[107]. In the text, Ayurveda outlined six tremors:

1. Vepathu (a generalized tremor)
2. Prevepana (excessive shaking)
3. Kampa vata (tremors because of vata)
4. Sirakampa (head tremor)
5. Spandin (quivering)
6. Kampana (tremors)

Number three on the list, Kampa vata, identified what we know today as Parkinson's disease.

Ayurveda's ancient history was perhaps the world's first genuine pooling of medical information and one of the earliest examples of networking. That they earn the distinction of first identifying Parkinson's is no surprise.

Almost eight centuries later, in 175 AD, Roman physician, surgeon, and philosopher Aelius Galenus[108] (Galen) described Parkinsonism as the "shaking palsy."

The modern Parkinson's research era[109] points to 1817 when James Parkinson published "An Essay on the Shaking Palsy[110]" and described the neurological disorder that Ayurveda, Galen, and others before identified and published material advancing the neurological disorder. However, the science world did not take serious notice of Dr. Parkinson's work until decades later, around mid nine nineteenth century, when the field of neurology was born.

Jean-Martin Charcot[111], known as the father of neurology, expanded James Parkinson's work, named the disorder after Parkinson, and separated Parkinson's disease from other neurological diseases such as multiple sclerosis. Whereas Charcot revived James Parkinson's work and named Parkinson's disease, he discovered several other diseases, including amyotrophic lateral sclerosis[112], Charcot's joint[113], and Charcot-Marie-tooth disease[114] (peroneal muscular atrophy).

Charcot also created the anatomo-clinical method[115] distinguishing clinical features and pathological changes in post-mortem.

Parkinson's disease (PD) prevalence

Parkinson's disease (PD) strikes more people than "multiple sclerosis (MS), muscular dystrophy (MD), and amyotrophic lateral sclerosis (ALS) combined[116]."

Parkinson's is the second most prevalent neurological disorder of aging behind Alzheimer's[117]. Along with Alzheimer's, epilepsy, multiple sclerosis, and stroke, Parkinson's disease is a common neurological disorder[118].

How many people have Parkinson's disease (PD)?

United States PD

About 60,000 Americans get Parkinson's every year, adding to the 1.2 million already suffering PD in the United States[119].

United Kingdom PD

One in 500, 127,000 British live with Parkinson's disease[120] (PD).

Canada PD

Like the UK, Parkinson's disease (PD) strikes one of 500 Canadians, and over 100,000 live with PD[121].

Australia PD

One of every 250 or 80,000 Australians live with Parkinson's disease[122] (PD).

Global PD

One million Americans and over 10 million people worldwide live with Parkinson's disease[123].

What causes Parkinson's disease?

Rogue a-synuclein protein causes Parkinson's related neurological damage in the substantia nigra, but what makes the typically beneficial protein dysfunctional?

The image below shows the substantia nigra region where PD atrophy is prevalent.

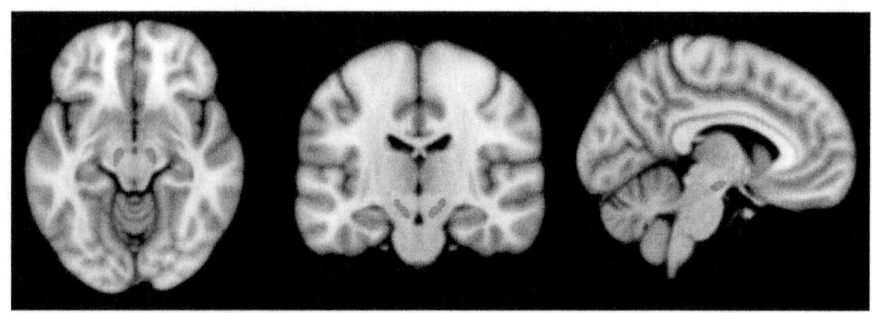

Substantia nigra[124] by (Zahang, Larcher, et al., 2017)

In the midbrain, substantia nigra atrophy is a core Parkinson's feature.

Genetics

Researchers believe genetics cause less than fifteen percent of Parkinson's disease[125] (PD), many of those in the early onset cases[126]. While hereditary factors play a role, other causes drive most PD cases. What causes the other 85-90 percent?

Other possible PD causes

Although they call for further studies, the National Health Services in the UK points to the following environmental toxins[127].

- Industrial Pollution
- Herbicides
- Pesticides
- Traffic pollution

Johns Hopkins also points to toxins, including pesticides, herbicides, MPTP, Agent Orange, metals, solvents, and organic pollutants as likely culprits[128].

Who does Parkinson's disease strike?

Whereas women are more likely to get most dementias than men, men are 1.5 times more likely than women to get Parkinson's disease. Although more prevalent among black women, Parkinson's attacks women less than men.

Who are the three highest risk groups?

Highest PDD Risk Groups

Although the reasons remain dubious, most dementia types discriminate. Dementias discriminate by picking on particular kinds of people. For Parkinson's, the three groups:

- Males
- Hispanics
- Whites

Parkinson's spares no group but strikes males, Hispanics, and whites in disproportionate numbers. Why different dementias target different people remains a mystery.

The opposite of Alzheimer's, men are 1.5 times more likely than women to get Parkinson's disease[129].

And, unlike some dementias, Parkinson's targets more white than black people. Hispanics and non-Hispanic whites lead Parkinson's incidents per 100,000, with Hispanics at 16.6 and non-Hispanic whites at 13.6, compared to 11.3% for Asians and 10.2% for black people[130].

What percentage of Parkinson's disease develops dementia?

Researchers calculate 50-80 percent of Parkinson's disease (PD) develop dementia[131]. Clinical criteria demand dementia symptoms before shifting PD diagnosis to Parkinson's disease dementia (PDD).

Once Parkinson's patients develop dementia symptoms, PDD becomes more like dementia with Lewy bodies (DLB) the more the cognitive symptoms develop.

Chapter 7: PARKINSON'S DISEASE DEMENTIA (PDD) SYMPTOMS

> *In this gait, the patient will have rigidity and bradykinesia. He or she {stoops} with the head and neck forward, with flexion at the knees. The whole upper extremity is also in flexion, with the fingers usually extended. The patient walks with slow little steps known as Marche a petits pas (walk of little steps). {The} patient may also have difficulty initiating steps. The patient may show an involuntary inclination to take accelerating steps, known as festination. This gait {is} in Parkinson's disease or any other condition causing parkinsonism, such as side effects from drugs.*
>
> *–Stanford Medicine*[132]

In the beginning, there is no dementia in Parkinson's disease, so whether it develops into Parkinson's disease dementia (PDD) or not, all cases begin as Parkinson's disease (PD). Dementia occurring first suggests dementia with Lewy bodies (DLB).

While not present at the time of Parkinson's disease diagnosis, for DLB, dementia symptoms eventually occur and prompt an updated diagnosis of Parkinson's disease dementia.

We will point out which symptoms likely occur first but include all the symptoms somebody with PDD might experience. Since no two cases are exact, the symptoms vary from one person to the next, depending on brain atrophy region and severity.

Motor symptoms

Parkinson's causes various motor problems, including balance and gait issues and bradykinesia (slow movements). PDD patients suffer from stiffness, and moving grows more complicated, including walking.

PDD patients' postures stoop. They often suffer tremors (involuntary twitching and movements).

Behavioral and Mood Symptoms

Parkinson's patients suffer various behavioral and mood problems, the most prevalent being anxiety and depression.

According to Anna Morenkova, MD, Ph.D., UCI School of Medicine's

Department of Neurology, PDD patients also undergo personality changes.

"A person who was always conscientious becomes careless," said Morenkova. "A previously easy-going person becomes rigid and stubborn. An outgoing social butterfly turns into a stay-at-home introvert."

Cognitive Issues

Cognitive issues include attention deficits, slower thinking, and decreased executive function. Parkinson's patients often struggle to find the correct word. Learning grows progressively more difficult because Parkinson's attacks the part of the brain responsible for remembering. PDD patients also suffer visuospatial dysfunction.

Sleep Symptoms

Parkinson's patients suffer several sleep problems, including **REM**, vivid nightmares, sleep fragmentation (continuous awakening), and sleep apnea.

The sleep issues compound the other Parkinson's symptoms, adding another layer of discomfort and anxiety.

Motor Symptoms

Most of us have seen people with Parkinson's disease. Michael J. Fox. Robin Williams. Muhammad Ali. Parkinson's struck all three famous men. Most see so many people with Parkinson's; they mistake other disorders for PD that share "Parkinson's-like" symptoms. Most of the Parkinson's symptoms we're familiar with are motor skills.

We watched Parkinson's take down one of the greatest athletes ever. A man who stood for work ethic, confidence, courage, toughness, yet words flowed from his tongue like the most significant poets and orators. Muhammad Ali fought the disease like the champ he was, but most of us cringed, watching his glorious body deteriorate until we only saw him in a wheelchair.

PDD motor symptoms

- Bradykinesia
- Gait/Walking problems
- Dystonia
- Rigidity
- Tremors
- Unstable posture

Other PDD Symptoms

- Constipation
- Dizziness or fainting
- Drooling

- Early satiety
- Fatigue
- Increased dandruff
- Lightheadedness
- Losing the sense of smell or taste
- Pain
- Sexual problems
- Urinary urgency, frequency, and incontinence
- Vision problems
- Weight loss

Parkinson's Symptoms Sources: European Parkinson's Disease Association[133], Alzheimer's Society[134], Parkinson's Foundation[135], The Lancet Neurology[136], *Parkinson's News Today*[137], EPDA[138], Parkinson's Foundation[139], LBDA[140]

II. FTD-RELATED DEMENTIAS

The series devotes books to two FTD-related dementias:
1. Behavioral Variant Frontotemporal Dementia
2. Progressive Supranuclear Palsy

The PPA subtypes also have FTD links, but we list them separately as PPA dementias.

Chapter 8: WHAT IS FRONTOTEMPORAL DEMENTIA?

Perhaps the fourth largest dementia category, frontotemporal dementia, does not receive the headlines nor research money as its more prevalent cousins: Alzheimer's, Vascular dementia, and Lewy body dementia.

FRONTOTEMPORAL DEMENTIA

Also called Pick's disease, frontotemporal dementia begins as frontotemporal degeneration (FTD) and progresses to dementia symptoms.

Frontotemporal dementia attacks the front and side sections of the brain. A steady, progressive disease, frontotemporal dementia, causes behavior changes and destroys the ability to process language.

To further define frontotemporal dementia, let's turn to other authorities.

Frontotemporal dementia affects "the frontal and temporal lobes of the brain (the front and sides) in particular." according to the National Health Service in the UK. "These parts of the brain {are} responsible for language and the ability to plan and organise and are important in controlling behaviour[141]."

The UCSF Weill Institute for Neurosciences describes FTD:

> *Frontotemporal dementia (FTD) is a group of related conditions resulting from the progressive degeneration of the temporal and frontal lobes of the brain. These areas of the brain play a significant role in decision-making, behavioral control, emotion and language*[142].

FTD produces contrasting symptoms depending on the neurological damage to the brain's frontal, temporal, and insular lobes. The divergence also explains why there are two primary subtypes.

According to the NIH, the brain's frontal lobes serves many purposes, including[143]:

- Censoring social behavior
- Managing emotional responses
- Processing language and communication

When the protein deposits form in the frontal lobes, depending on the exact location, the result is behavioral variant frontotemporal dementia or primary progressive aphasia.

Predominant symptoms including social behavior and emotional changes indicate behavioral variant frontotemporal dementia.

Neurological damage resulting in language and communication disorders suggests primary progressive aphasia.

As dementia develops and the deposits spread, the symptoms overlap between the two primary frontotemporal dementia types.

What Is the Difference Between FTD And FLTD?

Many view FTD and FLTD as synonymous. Are FTD and FLTD synonymous?

No.

Frontotemporal dementia (FTD) is a frontotemporal lobar degeneration (FTLD) subtype. According to Dr. E. Mohandas, Elite Mission Hospital, "Frontotemporal disorders are forms of dementia caused by a family of brain diseases known as frontotemporal lobar degeneration (FTLD)."

Just as frontotemporal dementia (FTD) is one of many dementias, FTD is one of several FLTD neurological disorders caused by damage to the frontal lobes.

Who does Frontotemporal Dementia Strike?

Genetics causes one-third of frontotemporal dementia[144].

Whereas women are more likely to have Alzheimer's, and men have Lewy body dementia, frontotemporal has no gender preference.

A study released in the *Journal of Neurology, Neurosurgery & Psychiatry* concluded that 3% of seniors over 85 suffer Frontotemporal dementia[145].

One key to dementias such as frontotemporal is discovering accurate urine or blood tests for early diagnosis. We do not know if the diagnosis is correct unless they perform an autopsy once the patient dies.

How many people have Frontotemporal Dementia (FTD)?

About 60,000 Americans suffer frontotemporal dementia, although the number would climb much higher if we had an accurate urine or blood test.

I view American numbers as dubious, as, like many global authorities, cannot provide more than a ballpark figure. The combination of misdiagnosis and faulty, time-delayed record-keeping leads to too many estimates and ridiculous ranges of possibilities.

As I harp in every dementia section, we need blood or urine tests to diagnose behavioral variant frontotemporal dementia (bvFTD) well before the first symptoms manifest. I am no more fond of repetition than you, but I repeat: *We do not know if the diagnosis is correct unless they perform an autopsy once the patient dies.*

FTD Percentage of Dementia

The Association of Frontotemporal Degeneration estimates FTD totals 10-20% of dementia[146]. However, Stanford Medical School claims FTD represents 2-10% of dementia cases[147]. Other reputed authorities estimate 2-20%, some towards the high and others the low end.

NIH and those who control medical research funding sometimes neglect bvFTD because other dementias such as Alzheimer's, Lewy body dementia, and vascular dementia strike more seniors 65 and older.

While the logic of devoting most research money to help most people is unmistakable, such thinking only works in theory and sometimes not at all in practice.

I want cures for disorders striking seniors, but challenge suggestions we should not devote research money to rarer diseases that disproportionately attack young people.

Early onset FTD Percentage

If we consider early onset dementia even more devastating than late-onset dementia, we must view bvFTD and the FTD-related dementias as significant.

Frontotemporal dementia strikes more people in their 40s than most dementias, accounting for over 20% of early onset dementia.

A *PubMed* study shows FTD accounts for 30.6% of early onset dementia[148]. Exact percentages vary, but experts agree FTD is the second-leading cause of early onset dementia, behind only Alzheimer's.

What Age Does Frontotemporal Dementia (FTD) Strike?

Most cases strike people between 40 and 65, although FTD inflicts people as young as 20 and in their eighties[149]. The average age for those diagnosed with frontotemporal dementia is age 57, 13 years younger than age 70 for other dementia patients[150].

"These disorders are among the most common dementias that strike at younger ages," according to John Hopkins Medicine. "Symptoms typically start between the ages of 40 and 65, but FTD can strike young adults and those who are older[151]."

What Causes Frontotemporal Dementia (FTD)?

Too often for dementias, the official answer within the medical community is the cause remains unknown, and this applies to frontotemporal dementia (FTD).

If science cannot name the exact cause, what do we know?

Genetics causes a third of FTD incidents. The number is higher than most dementias, except Down syndrome with Alzheimer's and Huntington's disease, for which genetics is 100% responsible.

However, this means two/thirds of FTD cases are not family related. Nor does having a parent with FTD a dementia sentence.

Frontotemporal dementia is a sporadic neurological disorder. According to the Association for Frontotemporal Degeneration, one is no more at risk for FTD if a parent has the disorder than if they do not[152].

"Researchers have linked certain subtypes of FTD to mutations on several genes," per the University of Rochester Medical Center. "Some people with FTD have tiny structures, called Pick bodies, in their brain cells. Pick bodies have an abnormal amount or type of protein[153]."

Frontotemporal dementia manifests by damaging brain cells in the brain's frontal and temporal lobes.

Frontotemporal dementia (FTD) symptoms

In the image below, we are interested in the Frontal lobe and the Temporal lobe regions, the front and sides of the brain.

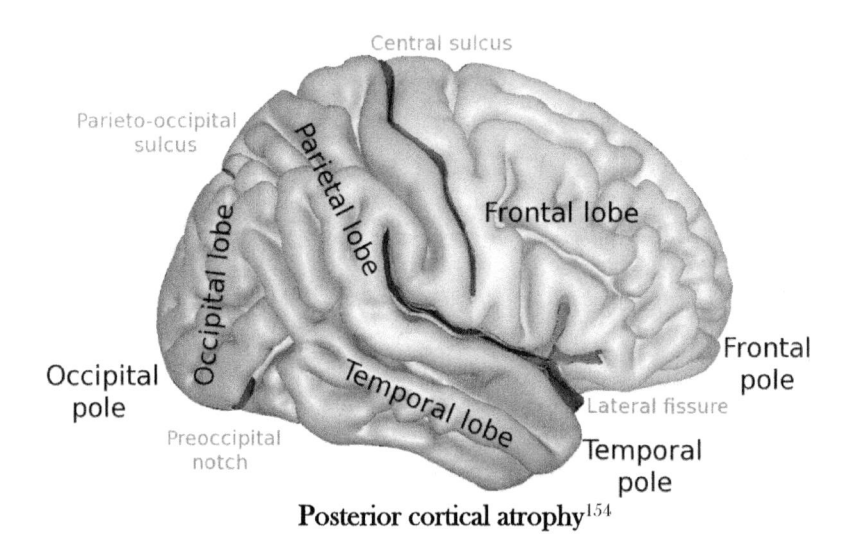

Posterior cortical atrophy[154]

While science must determine the risk factors and causes, we know much more about the symptoms of frontotemporal dementias:

- Behavioral changes[155]
- Change in eating habits, including eating much more, liking foods you always hated before[156]
- Deterioration of personal hygiene[157]
- Diminished vocabulary[158]
- Distracted easier and more often than usual[159]
- Irritated over trivial matters[160]
- Growing dependence[161]
- Impaired judgment[162]
- Inarticulate[163]
- Incapable of abstract thought[164]
- Inflexible thinking[165]
- Lacks compassion and empathy[166]

- Less conversational[167]
- Less enthusiastic[168]
- Memory issues[169] (advanced stages)
- Muscle spasms[170]
- Misuses words, such as referring to plates as spoons, or dogs as cats[171]
- Mood changes[172]
- More withdrawn and secluded than usual[173]
- Needs reminders to do basic daily tasks[174]
- Nervous and obsessive behavior, which includes rubbing hands, tapping feet, pacing the same stretch, mumbling or humming[175] that didn't exist before[176]
- Deteriorating organizational skills[177]
- Repeats exact phrases over and over like stuck in a loop[178]
- Repeats what other people say[179]
- Rude behavior considered out of character[180]
- Uninhibited[181]

Let's break the symptoms down by category.

Two FTD-related Dementia Types

There are two FTD-associated dementias.

1. Behavior-variant frontotemporal dementia (bvFTD)
2. Progressive supranuclear palsy (PSP)

The former causes behavioral changes while the latter attacks language skills. Behavior-variant first destroys emotion, while progressive supranuclear palsy (PSP) attacks motor skills.

According to *Neuroscience Research Australia*, "When the initial damage is in the frontal lobe (called behavioral-variant FTD), the main changes are in personality and behaviour. Individuals with damage predominantly in the temporal lobe (either progressive non-fluent aphasia or semantic dementia) lose the ability to speak or understand language[182]."

We discuss the PPA subtypes separately, so let's focus on behavioral variant frontotemporal dementia (bvFTD) and progressive supranuclear palsy (PSP).

Chapter 9: bvFTD BEHAVIORAL VARIANT FRONTOTEMPORAL DEMENTIA?

Sometimes called Pick's disease, frontotemporal dementia begins as frontotemporal degeneration (FTD) and progresses to dementia symptoms.

Frontotemporal dementia attacks the front and side sections of the brain. A steady, progressive disease, frontotemporal dementia causes behavior changes (problems) and destroys the ability to process language.

To further define frontotemporal dementia, let's turn to other authorities.

Frontotemporal dementia affects "the frontal and temporal lobes of the brain (the front and sides) in particular," according to the National Health Service in the UK. "These parts of the brain are {responsible} for language and the ability to plan and organise, and are important in controlling behaviour[183]."

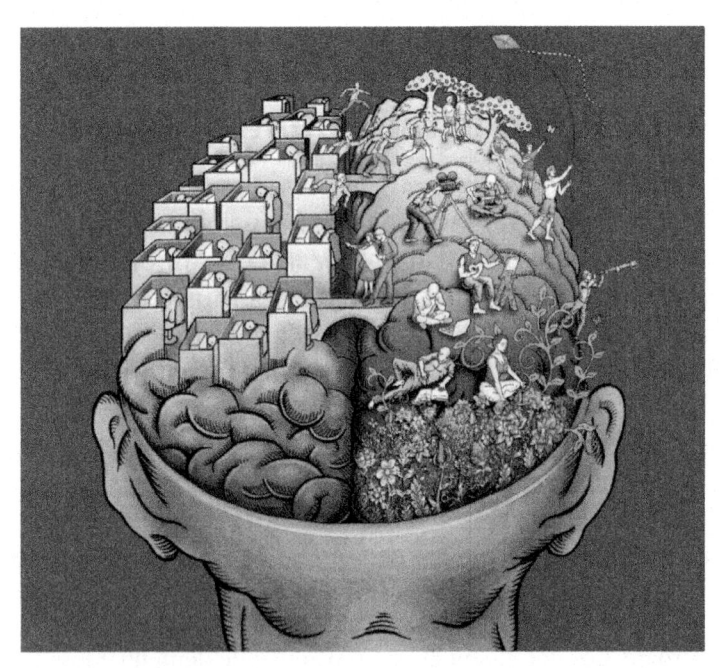

Right Brain[184]

Frontotemporal dementia stands out in a few ways. Genetics causes a third of incidents.

bvFTD strikes most people between ages 45 and 65, although it inflicts people as young as 20 and in their eighties[185]. The average age for those diagnosed with frontotemporal dementia is age 57, 13 years younger than age 70 for other dementia patients[186].

Frontotemporal dementia manifests by damaging brain cells in the brain's frontal and temporal lobes.

According to *Neuroscience Research Australia*, "When the initial damage is in the frontal lobe (called behavioral-variant FTD), the main changes are in personality and behavior[187]."

Behavioral-variant frontotemporal dementia Prevalence

The most prevalent frontotemporal dementia, bvFTD, accounts for 50-70% of cases within the FTD family. If the 20% gap in possibilities gives pause, join the club.

Getting an exact number of FTD cases is impossible.

bvFTD Symptoms

To make it easier to grasp, we divide the symptoms into behavioral, cognitive, and others.

Behavioral Symptoms

- Personality changes[188]
- Mood swings[189]
- More withdrawn and secluded than usual[190]
- Nervous and obsessive behavior, which includes rubbing hands, tapping feet, pacing the same stretch, mumbling or humming[191] that didn't exist before[192]
- Rude behavior considered out of character[193]
- Uninhibited[194]
- Irritated over trivial matters[195]
- Inflexible thinking[196]
- Lacks compassion and empathy[197]
- Less enthusiastic[198]

We associate the above symptoms with behavioral variant frontotemporal dementia (bvFTD) and are not the victim's fault. The neurological disorder causes a person to act out of character because of neuron damage in the brain's area responsible for censoring and processing thoughts required to behave according to societal norms.

Next, let's examine cognitive symptoms.

Cognitive Symptoms

- Needs reminders to do basic daily tasks[199]
- Distracted easier and more often than usual[200]
- Impaired judgment[201]
- Incapable of abstract thought[202]

- Growing dependence[203]
- Deteriorating organizational skills[204]
- Memory issues[205] (advanced stages)

Cognitive symptoms somewhat resemble Alzheimer's, often causing misdiagnosis. Documenting full symptoms helps doctors order the correct tests and reduce the odds of misdiagnosing bvFTD for one of the other prominent dementias.

As frontotemporal dementia advances, it becomes less distinguishable from Alzheimer's. In the late stage, most dementia types resemble each other because damage to the brain spreads.

With no FTD test, doctors must diagnose the disorder through elimination.

Let's move to other symptoms.

Other Symptoms

- Change in eating habits, including eating much more, liking foods you always hated before[206]
- Deterioration of personal hygiene[207]

These symptoms are problematic for both frontotemporal dementia subtypes.

If you notice several uncharacteristic behaviors from the list in you or a loved one, see a neurologist at once. Document the symptoms you're experiencing to enhance your physician's diagnosis.

No two patients develop exact frontotemporal dementia symptoms, as bvFTD uniquely strikes each. The slightest difference where FTD first attacks the brain produces various symptoms. The symptoms develop once somebody gets frontotemporal dementia depending on the brain area affected and how rapidly the bvFTD attacks are.

When the listed symptoms appear, you or your loved one cannot see a competent doctor fast enough. While the medical community possesses no cures in their bag of tools, they can treat and slow symptoms, extending the quality of life.

Until we find a cure, individuals must focus on preventing or slowing dementia. The medical community must treat symptoms with drugs and help the patient through physical, speech, and occupational therapy.

Instead of panicking, which is natural, the diagnosed and family must pull themselves together and do what they can to make the most of the remaining quality time.

The person diagnosed and their loved ones must ask: **What is one more day, week, month, or year of quality time worth?**

I am not suggesting anybody neglect the many burdens the diagnosis brings on an individual and their closest loved ones.

Address future concerns, financial and otherwise. Create a Living Will, provide a trustworthy person the Power of Attorney, and get out in front of the coming storm while you can.

Figure out who will care for you or a loved one when daily help becomes necessary. Understand such caregiving becomes a 24/7 job down the stretch.

The mentioned tasks and other steps are priorities, but prioritize extending the quality of life as long as possible. When we remove the medical, legal, and economic decisions, the most important thing is for everybody concerned to overcome the shock, hurt, and pain.

The symptoms are not usually severe enough to prevent somebody from carrying on much as usual in the early stages. The challenge for you and your loved ones is to enjoy life while possible. Instead of dreading the coming storm, embrace the remaining possibilities.

According to the Penn Frontotemporal degeneration Center, bvFTD shows "progressive atrophy (cell loss) in frontal and anterior temporal regions of the brain leading to alterations in complex thinking, personality, and behavior[208]."

The behavioral changes hurt family, friends, and associates. However, bvFTD patients suffer a wide range of emotional and behavioral disorders. While some behavior is unacceptable and loved ones and caregivers must help manage, the bvFTD patient has little or no control.

The UCSF Memory and Aging Center describes behavioral variant frontotemporal dementia.

> *People with behavioral variant frontotemporal dementia (bvFTD) often have trouble controlling their behavior. They may say inappropriate things or ignore other peoples' feelings. bvFTD may affect how a person deals with everyday situations. bvFTD can also affect language or thinking skills. Unfortunately, people with bvFTD rarely notice these changes[209].*

Perhaps the most troubling aspect of the quote is the last sentence. The disease already chips away at the person's personality, but the victim remains oblivious.

The point illustrates the importance of loved ones monitoring each other's behavior.

bvFTD Recap

From the introduction, we know that frontotemporal dementia (FTD) attacks the front and sides of the brain and the frontal and temporal lobes. The frontal and temporal lobes play significant roles in language, organizing, and behavior.

There are two types of FTD and primary progressive aphasia.

Other points to take from this section:

- 60,000 Americans suffer FTD

- There is no accurate test
- Doctors often misdiagnose FTD for Alzheimer's or other diseases
- FTD is one of the most prevalent dementias to strike people in their 40s or 50s in their prime

While behavioral variant frontotemporal dementia (bvFTD) represents most FTD cases, some develop multiple types. A person can also develop Alzheimer's or another dementia along with FTD, classified as mixed dementia.

Chapter 10: WHAT IS PROGRESSIVE SUPRANUCLEAR PALSY (PSP)?

Progressive means continuous severity. *Supranuclear* refers to the lesion cortical or superior to the brain's nucleus. *Palsy* suggests weakness or paralysis, often associated with involuntary tremors.

S*upranuclear palsy* causes weakness or paralysis on one side of the body.

Also called Steele-Richardson-Olszewski syndrome, progressive supranuclear palsy is a neurological disorder that exhibits Parkinsonism symptoms such as balance, walking, speech, and other symptoms we soon discuss in greater detail.

In 1964, three scientists—John Steel, J. Clifford Richardson, and Jerzy Olszewski—published a study showing a divergence from typical Parkinson's disease.

Some still refer to their discovery as the Steel-Richardson-Olszewski syndrome, but most refer to the disorder as progressive supranuclear palsy.

Until 1964, neurologists recognized a case now and then but lumped them with Parkinson's disease. However, cut the doctors some slack as PSP and PD share several Parkinsonism symptoms, and no PSP category existed.

Not to excuse incompetence, but the best doctors also make mistakes with such limited tools. We cannot prevent dementia misdiagnosis by weeding out incompetent doctors. While the medical professional should weed out the unethical and incompetent, that alone will not prevent dementia misdiagnosis. We expect the impossible until we arm doctors with accurate blood or urine tests for each dementia.

Is there a PSP Cure?

As with most dementia-related diseases, there is no cure.

Diagnosing PSP poses challenges, leading to misdiagnoses or late diagnoses. A delayed diagnosis means delayed treatment, and misdiagnosis risks the wrong treatment. A late start and limited options stymie efforts to slow progression, making it essential to improve and speed diagnosis, allowing treatment options a better chance of slowing PSP.

Early diagnosis is the key if we ever reverse PSP and other dementias. When the symptoms manifest and medical officials diagnose, the neuro damage is already significant. I'm uncertain future medicine will ever reverse once a certain amount of neurological damage occurs.

We need more significant investment into PSP and other dementias to develop blood or urine testing to detect the dementia years or decades before symptoms arise and cures for the underlying causes. We likely can only defeat dementia in the prodromal stage, an impossibility without the blood or urine tests I keep harping.

PSP Life Expectancy

Although not considered fatal, several later-stage PSP symptoms cause death, including choking, injuries, and pneumonia.

According to the NHS, the expected average PSP life range is 6-10 years from when the symptoms manifest.

How Many People Get Progressive Supranuclear Palsy (PSP)?

NIH estimates progressive supranuclear palsy inflicts six of every 100,000 people worldwide and that 20,000 Americans live with PSP[210].

According to ASCE Neuron, PSP represents 1% of dementia[211].

Who Is Most Likely to Get Progressive Supranuclear Palsy (PSP)?

Progressive supranuclear palsy (PSP) attacks people over 60 more significantly than younger people. PSP also attacks men more often than women.

Medscape claims most people get PSP in their 50s and 60s, and the symptoms manifest a third of the time for people under sixty[212].

There is no genetic or family link in most PSP cases, although science links it to an abnormal tau protein buildup.

How Does Progressive Supranuclear Palsy (PSP) Differ from Parkinson's' Disease?

While PSP and PD share several symptoms, progressive supranuclear palsy differs from Parkinson's in several ways.

Progressive supranuclear palsy progresses faster than Parkinson's disease (PD).

Whereas Parkinson's patients often tilt their heads forward, somebody with PSP is more likely to tilt theirs backward. Eye movements remain normal in most PD patients but are abnormal in progressive supranuclear palsy patients. Swallowing and speech are more severe in PSP than PD, and PSP often spares patients the Parkinson's associated tremors[213].

Progressive Supranuclear Palsy Causes

Common for dementia and other neurological disorders, we do not yet know the exact cause of progressive supranuclear palsy (PSP). Science, however, links the rogue PSP-related protein, tau[214].

If you've read much about Alzheimer's, you know about protein tau and the associated tangles. The MAPT gene in chromosome 17q21 produces tau[215].

TAU the Superhero

The tau family has a high-soluble microtubule-related protein and six isoforms, including 352-441 amino acids.

Regarding neurological disorders, protein is a superhero-turned villain. As superheroes, tau plays a vital role in the central nervous system by regulating the axonal transport of vesicles and stabilizing microtubules.

TAU Turned Villain

What causes the tau to turn rogue remains a mystery, but there is a pattern. Essential protein turns abnormal and attacks the very structure it once built, maintained, or protected.

ASCE NEURON explains progressive supranuclear palsy:

> The hallmark of PSP is the accumulation of abnormal deposits of the protein tau in nerve cells in the brain so that the cells do not function properly and eventually die. The appearance of deposits of the microtubule-associated tau protein termed 'neurofibrillary tangles' is a common feature of tauopathies {shared} with Alzheimer's disease. These neuronal tau deposits are {a} primary driver of neurodegeneration[216].

Rogue tau protein causes 30-40% of Alzheimer's disease and links to a few other dementias, including progressive supranuclear palsy (**PSP**).

PSP Cortical fibrillary Tangles

Although found in the spinal cord and central cortex, globose neurofibrillary tangles are more prevalent in the subcortical areas. PSP neurodegeneration occurs in the basal ganglia.

Progressive supranuclear palsy symptoms

Progressive supranuclear palsy causes a wide range of behavior and mood problems. As with any neurological disorder causing behavior issues, this can be difficult for loved ones and caregivers.

However, you must remember the behavior is not the person's fault, but a neurological disorder destroys part of their mind. It often involves the frontal and temporal lobes with behavior and mood problems, explaining why progressive supranuclear palsy lists in the frontotemporal degeneration family.

However, PSP-related symptoms go well beyond the associated mood and behavior disorders, including a devastating attack on motor skills and muscle control.

NIH describes progressive supranuclear palsy symptoms.

> *The pattern of signs and symptoms can {differ} from*

person to person. The most frequent first symptom of PSP is a loss of balance while walking. Individuals may have unexplained falls or a stiffness and awkwardness in gait.

As the disease progresses, most people will {develop} a blurring of vision and problems controlling eye movement. In fact, eye problems, in particular slowness of eye movements, usually offer the first definitive clue that PSP is the proper diagnosis. Individuals affected by PSP especially have trouble voluntarily shifting their gaze vertically (i.e., downward and/or upward) and also can have trouble controlling their eyelids. This can lead to a need to move the head to look in different directions, involuntary closing of the eyes, prolonged or infrequent blinking, or difficulty in opening the eyes.

As NIH illustrates, progressive supranuclear palsy produces a wide range of symptoms. The symptoms start as young as forty, but not until the early sixties for most PSP patients.

To some extent, progressive supranuclear palsy combines Parkinson's and behavioral frontotemporal dementia, attacking both the mind and the body.

Let's list the most common earlier stage symptoms.

PSP symptoms list

Progressive supranuclear palsy symptoms include:

- Apathetic
- Balance issues
- Behavior changes (reckless and flawed decision-making)
- Blurred or double vision
- Falling (often backward)
- Irritable
- Major fatigue
- Moody
- Muscles discomfort
- Neck stiffness
- Personality changes
- Photophobia (bright lights sensitivity)
- Trouble looking up or down

PSP Symptoms Sources: National Health Service[217], National Institute of Neurological Disorders and Stroke[218]

We discuss progressive supranuclear palsy symptoms more in the symptoms section.

III. PRIMARY PROGRESSIVE APHASIA

We cover two primary progressive aphasia (PPA) types in the book series. One is Alzheimer's dominant, and the other is FTD dominant, although AD and FTD play roles in both PPA varieties.

Two PPA types:

1. Nonfluent/agrammatic variant of primary progressive aphasia (naPPA)
2. Logopenic Progressive Aphasia (LPA)

Chapter 11: WHAT IS PRIMARY PROGRESSIVE APHASIA (PPA)?

Depending on the pathology, primary progressive aphasia is Alzheimer's-related or FTD-related. FTD is most linked to two subtypes, while Alzheimer's is predominant in the third. However, both Alzheimer's and FTD play a role in all three subtypes.

Mesulam Center for Cognitive Neurology and Alzheimer's Disease defines primary progressive aphasia:

> *Adults of any age can develop primary progressive aphasia (PPA), but it is more common in people under the age of 65. Individuals with PPA may have difficulties in word-finding, word usage, word order, word comprehension or word spelling. Other thinking skills (including memory for recent events, spatial orientation, recognizing faces and the essential features of personality) are initially preserved. The symptoms of PPA can cause limitations in professional, social and recreational activities that may affect one's overall quality of life[219].*

An appropriate description. However, the last sentence might be an understatement of the century.

Let's compare the Mesulam description with one from Northwestern Medicine.

> *Primary progressive aphasia (PPA) is a form of cognitive impairment that involves a progressive loss of language function. Language is a uniquely human faculty that allows us to communicate with each other through the use of words.*
>
> *Our language functions include speaking, understanding what others are saying, repeating things we have heard, naming common objects, reading and writing. Aphasia is a general term used to refer to deficits in language functions. PPA is caused by degeneration in the parts of the brain {responsible} for speech and language.*

We've viewed how notable organizations describe **PPA**. While speech and communication are central components to **PPA**, patients also suffer a severe cognitive decline as the disorder progresses.

An interesting characteristic of primary progressive aphasia (PPA) is one's word production increases before deteriorating, meaning loved ones and associates will not suspect a problem.

If a loved one remains oblivious, frontotemporal dementia develops undiagnosed, and the symptoms go unaddressed.

Let's next view the three PPA subtypes.

There are three primary progressive aphasia (PPA) types

1. Logopenic progressive aphasia (LPA)
2. Nonfluent-agrammatic variant primary progressive aphasia (naPPA)
3. Semantic variant primary progressive aphasia (svPPA)

The three PPA types[220] cause different symptoms, which we discuss in the next section. We devote a chapter to each subtype once we finish our general PPA discussion.

Primary Progressive Aphasia (PPA) Causes

Pinpointing the causes for most dementias, including FTD, confounds science.

Genetics causes one-third of frontotemporal dementia. Whereas brain injuries or strokes cause most aphasia, Alzheimer's or frontotemporal degeneration causes primary progressive aphasia.

According to the National Aphasia Association[221]:

> *PPA is caused by neurodegenerative diseases, such as Alzheimer's Disease or Frontotemporal Lobar Degeneration. PPA results from deterioration of brain tissue important for speech and language. Although the first symptoms are problems with speech and language, other problems associated with the underlying disease, such as memory loss, often occur later. PPA commonly begins as a subtle disorder of language, progressing to a nearly total inability to speak, in its most severe stage. The type or pattern of the language deficit may differ from patient to patient. The initial language disturbance may be fluent aphasia (i.e., the person may have normal or even increased rate of word production) or non-fluent aphasia (speech becomes effortful and the person produces fewer words). A less common variety begins with impaired word-finding and progressive deterioration of naming and comprehension, with relatively preserved articulation.*

Both Alzheimer's and frontotemporal dementia cause primary progressive aphasia (PPA), distinguishing it from other neurological diseases and explaining why doctors often confuse the latter for the former.

Since years ago including frontotemporal dementia in one of my books, I have called on the government to fund frontotemporal dementia research better. We need more research in three areas: causes, accurate and inexpensive tests, and a cure.

FTD researchers trudge along because most dementia research money goes to Alzheimer's, vascular dementia, and Lewy body dementia. I am not suggesting the top three dementias receive too much funding. They do not get enough research money, but far more than frontotemporal dementia.

Science tells us genetics causes a third of frontotemporal dementia cases, but we know too little concerning the other two-thirds.

FTLD-TDP, FTLD-tau, & Alzheimer's Disease

Science does not know the exact cause, but researchers have identified three pathologies associated to varying degrees with each PPA subtype.

FTLD stands for frontotemporal lobar degenerations. In frontotemporal dementia discussions, we focus on FTLD-TDP (TDP-43) and FTLD-tau.

The three primary progressive aphasia pathologies:

1. FTLD-TDP (TDP-43)
2. FTLD-tau
3. Alzheimer's Disease

Understanding PPA subtypes, it is vital to grasp a basic understanding of the three causes.

Since the media and science cover Alzheimer's more than the other dementias combined, I presume everybody has basic knowledge. Therefore, let's focus on FTLD-TDP and FTLD-tau.

What is FTLD-TDP (TDP-43)?

When discussing Alzheimer's, LATE, or other dementias, the topic turns to protein buildup, plaques, tangles, and similar descriptions.

Like the other proteins, TDP-43 serves a vital function. However, scientists do not understand, causes the protein to build up in clumps, killing brain cells and tissue.

What is TDP-43's normal function?

In the cell nucleus, TDP-43 binds to DNA, regulates transcription, starting the first step in protein production.

The Genetics Home Reference[222] describes TDP-43.

> *This protein can also bind to RNA, a chemical cousin of DNA, to ensure the RNA's stability. The TDP-43 protein*

> *{processes} molecules called messenger RNA (mRNA), which serve as the genetic blueprints for making proteins. By cutting and rearranging mRNA molecules in different ways, the TDP-43 protein controls the production of different versions of certain proteins. This process {called} alternative splicing. The TDP-43 protein can influence various functions of a cell by regulating protein production.*
>
> *The TARDBP gene {is} active (expressed) during early development before birth when new tissues are forming. Many of the proteins whose production is influenced by the TDP-43 protein are involved in nervous system and organ development.*

Genetics accounts for 20-40% of FTLD-TDP (TDP-43)[223].

TDP-43 serves a vital role in our development and health, so why is it implicated in dementia?

What goes wrong?

When TDP-43 misfold, it causes impaired thinking and memory loss[224].

What is FTLD-tau?

Proteins are essential to brain health but devastating when something mysterious goes wrong and turns them into the neuron and syntax killers linked to dementia.

When healthy, tau performs an essential role in the microtubules responsible for cells communicating with each other. Healthy tau stabilizes the microtubules, whereas unstable tau sticks and forms deposits and damages the microtubules[225].

The medical community divides FTLD-tau into four subtypes:
1. Argyrophilic Corticobasal degeneration (CBD)
2. Globular glial tauopathy (GGT)
3. Progressive supranuclear palsy (PSP)
4. Pick's disease.

FTLD-tau represents one primary progressive aphasia pathology.

"Tau (the Greek letter) is a microtubule associated protein, encoded by the MAPT gene on 17q21," said Dimitri P Agamanolis, MD, from *Neuropathology*. "Normally, {phosphorylated}, tau is present mainly in axons where it binds and stabilizes microtubules. In FTLDs, abnormal deposits of hyperphosphorylated tau (paired helical or straight filaments) {deposit} in neurons and glial cells[226]."

The question science must answer: What destabilizes the tau protein? Is the initial problem the protein or something else?

Some neurologists such as Dale Bredesen and David Perlmutter argue the zealous focus on protein rather than the actual causes is why every dementia drug trial fails. Although they are fighting the current, such neurologists argue protein buildups are protective responses, not the reason.

Chapter 12: NONFLUENT/AGRAMMATICAL VARIANT OF PRIMARY PROGRESSIVE APHASIA (naPPA)

Also called progressive non-fluent aphasia (PNFA) shares similarities with the other two PPAs but distinguishes itself by how it attacks.

This frustrating primary progressive aphasia subtype inhibits people from saying words they know, words on the tip of their tongue. Patients also struggle to form sentences in the correct word or grammatical order.

The speech mechanism breaks down in this grammatic disorder. In most cases, tau protein buildup in the brain's anterior superior and inferior frontal-temporal sections causes neurodegeneration.

Nonfluent-agrammatic variant primary progressive aphasia (naPPA) Causes

Also called progressive non-fluent aphasia (PNFA), nonfluent-agrammatic variant primary aphasia (naPPA) accounts for up to 30 percent of FTD.

According to the Penn FTD Center[227], misfolded tau protein buildup in gray matter neurons causes almost 70% of non-fluent-agrammatic variant primary progressive aphasia (naPPA).

Genetics cause protein TDP-43 buildup responsible for non-fluent-agrammatic variant primary progressive aphasia.

According to Grossman, the pathology of naPPA takes four paths[228].

- 52%   FTLD-tau
- 25%   Alzheimer's disease
- 19%   FTLD-TDP
- 4%   Other

Whereas FTLD-tau plays a minor role in lvPPA, it is the dominant pathology for naPPA. Alzheimer's plays a lesser but significant role, accounting for a quarter of all cases. The opposite of lvPPA, FTLD-TDP plays a more secondary role, accounting for 19% of naPPA.

naPPA Life Expectancy

According to the UCSF, the average naPPA patient lives 8-10 years once symptoms begin[229].

Who is Most Likely to get naPPA?

Another dementia that strikes people in their prime, naPPA strikes most people before age sixty.

Nonfluent-agrammatic variant primary progressive aphasia (naPPA) symptoms

Grammar, motor skills, and sentence comprehension are more common in nonfluent-agrammatic variant primary progressive aphasia (nfvPPA).

- Pronunciation problems
- Reduced object recognition
- Slow, broken speech
- Speech requires greater effort
- Syntactic impairment
- Word comprehension impairment
- Unusual grammar problems

Let's discuss the symptoms more in the stages section.

Chapter 13: LOGOPENIC PROGRESSIVE APHASIA (LPA)

Also called Logopenic primary progressive aphasia and Logopenic variant PPA, logopenic progressive aphasia (LPA) is a primary progressive aphasia subtype. Both Alzheimer's and FTD cause LPA, but we list it as an Alzheimer's subtype because AD causes most LPA cases.

Unlike other primary progressive aphasias, LPA's pathology, including amyloid deposits and neurofibrillary tangles, resembles Alzheimer's.

LPA begins with sporadic speech deficits and trouble finding the correct word. Sentence comprehension deteriorates[230]. Somebody with LPA understands words and their meaning, but neuron damage makes it impossible for them to move the muscles responsible for speech. As symptoms manifest, grammar deteriorates, including wrong pronouns, verb tenses, and word order.

The more difficult speech becomes, one withdraws or shortens sentences, leaving words out altogether. Instead of saying: "Tomorrow is my son's birthday," they say: "Son birthday... Tomorrow."

Logopenic Progressive Aphasia (LPA) Causes

What causes logopenic progressive aphasia (LPA) remains unknown. Researchers point to amyloid and tau protein accumulations in the brain like Alzheimer's, which kills brain cells and inferior parietal lobe and posterior temporal cortex shrinkage[231].

Three primary causes of Logopenic progressive aphasia (LPA)

According to Murray Grossman, Department of Neurology, University of Pennsylvania, LPA's pathology takes three paths[232].

- 50% Alzheimer's disease
- 38% FTLD-TDP
- 12% FTLD-tau

In LPA, Alzheimer's causes half of the cases, while FTLD-TDP causes 38% and FTLD-tau only 12% of incidents.

Who is Most Likely to get LPA?

LPA inflicts people in their 30s or 70s, but the average age is fifty. Somebody with Alzheimer's disease lives with a higher risk of logopenic progressive aphasia (LPA) than somebody without AD.

Logopenic progressive aphasia (LPA) Symptoms

Logopenic progressive aphasia (LPA) symptoms include word and phrase repetition, trouble finding the correct word, sentence, word comprehension,

spelling, and reading.
- Grammar decline
- Impaired speech sound
- Impaired object knowledge
- Inability to comprehend or remember words
- Repeating words, phrases, and sentences
- Trouble finding the correct word

We will discuss these symptoms more in the stages section. First, let's list the symptoms for the other two subtypes.

Chapter 14: SEMANTIC PRIMARY PROGRESSIVE APHASIA (sPPA)

The third PPA strips the ability to recognize single words. People suffering semantic variant primary progressive aphasia (sPPA) often cannot identify intimate faces or familiar objects[233].

They cannot answer what a remote control is and know not how to search for one. Hand them the remote, however, and they recognize and understand.

Somebody with sPPA uses a lot of filler words. Instead of saying, "I'm going to the kitchen," they might say: "I'm going in that there place."

Semantic variant primary progressive aphasia (sPPA) Causes

Scientists struggle to understand semantic variant primary progressive aphasia (svPPA) but confirm protein TDP-43 in the temporal lobes brain regions[234] responsible for language skills[235].

Dr. Grossman names three sPPA pathologies[236]:
69% FTLD-TDP
25% Alzheimer's disease
6% FTLD-tau

Unlike lvFTD and naPPA, FTLD-TDP accounts for 69% of sPPA. FTLD-tau only accounts for 6% of cases, while Alzheimer's accounts for a quarter of sPPA.

The same three pathologies cause all three subtypes, but to varying degrees. While scientists debate what causes the protein deposits and tangles, they agree the rogue protein kills the neurons.

The medical community has investigated dementia causes for decades and only found clues, creating enormous frustration and fierce debates.

sPPA Life Expectancy

According to UCSF, once diagnosed with sPPA, a person lives an average of 12 years[237].

Who is Most Likely to get svPPA?

Like other subtypes, sPPA attacks most people in their 50s and strikes younger and older.

Semantic Primary Progressive Aphasia (sPPA) Symptoms

Semantic primary progressive aphasia (sPPA) impairment includes word recognition, spelling, reading, people, objects, and single-word recognition.

sPPA symptoms:

- Can no longer grasp day-to-day things
- Declined object recognition
- Impaired person recognition
- Loses the ability to follow conversations
- No longer understands word meanings
- Reading decline
- Severe grammar decline
- Writing decline

PPA Symptom Sources:
Penn Frontotemporal Degeneration Center[238]
PubMed[239]
PubMed[240]
PubMed[241]

Primary Progressive Aphasia (PPA) Symptoms Comparison

Let's compare the symptoms between the three PPA subtypes.

LANGUAGE SKILLS & COGNITIVE SYMPTOMS	LPA	nPPA	sPPA
Cannot grasp day-to-day things	X		X
Forgets familiar words	X		
Comprehension problems	X		
Grammar decline	X	X	
Impaired object knowledge	X	X	
Impaired person recognition			X
Impaired speech sound	X		
Pronunciation problems		X	
Repeats words and phrases	X		
Slow, broken speech		X	
Speech requires great effort		X	
Speech sound decline	X		

Struggles to find the correct word	X		
Syntactic impairment		X	
Word comprehension problems	X	X	
Word meaning decline			X
Writing decline			X

LPA = Logopenic progressive aphasia
nPPA = nonfluent-agrammatic variant primary progressive aphasia
sPPA = Semantic variant primary progressive aphasia

The three primary progressive aphasia (PPA) subtypes produce a variety of primarily contrasting symptoms.

IV. VASCULAR RELATED DEMENTIAS

This section includes two vascular dementia categories. We show vascular dementia's similarities and dissimilarities.

1. Cortical vascular dementia
2. Subcortical vascular dementia/Binswanger disease

The section views the pathology of both vascular dementia categories. It also covers two cortical subtypes: Post-stroke dementia and multi-infarct dementia.

What causes cortical vascular dementia and Binswanger disease? How are they similar? Different? Is there a cure? We answer these and related questions in this section.

Chapter 15: WHAT IS VASCULAR-DEMENTIA?

Like dementia, vascular dementia is not a singular disease but several syndromes attributed to preventable vascular mechanisms[242].

The American Psychiatric divides vascular neurocognitive disorder into mild and major, depending on how much the medical condition disrupts daily life[243].

Diagnosing vascular dementia, like most dementia, is complex, and doctors often misdiagnose confusing it with Alzheimer's, which shares many similar symptoms.

According to an Institute of Clinical Neurobiology autopsy study released in *PubMed*, 50% of dementia-related deaths share Alzheimer's and vascular dementia[244]. The medical community calls it "mixed dementia" when over one dementia is present.

The National Institute on Aging describes vascular dementia[245]:

> *Vascular dementia, the second most common form of dementia in older adults after Alzheimer's disease and vascular cognitive impairment (VCI), result from injuries to vessels that supply blood to the brain, often after a stroke or series of strokes. The symptoms of vascular dementia can be {like} those of Alzheimer's, and both conditions can occur at the same time (a condition called "mixed dementia"). Symptoms of vascular dementia and VCI can begin suddenly and worsen or improve.*

Vascular Dementia Causes

Perhaps more than anything else, what makes each vascular subtype necessary is pathology. Each subtype is vascular dementia, much like California and New York are two states within a larger union.

Like the mentioned US States, the vascular dementias differ from each other, experiencing different pathways, histories, and results.

We discuss vascular dementia causes in a general sense, then scrutinize each subtype.

Vascular Dementia versus AD

Because the other dementias share similar symptoms, and there are no blood or urine tests, doctors often misdiagnose other dementias for Alzheimer's. Further complicating matters, there are several Alzheimer's subtypes, two dementia with Lewy bodies, two frontotemporal types, and three vascular dementias.

While doctors often confuse vascular dementia with Alzheimer's disease, there are apparent differences.

The University of California, San Francisco Memory, and Aging Center describes vascular dementia and how it differs from Alzheimer's disease.

> *The term vascular dementia (VD) is usually reserved for a subtly progressive worsening of memory and other cognitive functions {presumed caused by} vascular disease within the brain. VD patients often present with similar symptoms to Alzheimer's disease (AD) patients, however, the related changes in the brain are not {caused by} AD pathology but to chronic reduced blood flow in the brain, eventually resulting in dementia. Clinically, such patients can look very similar to patients with AD, and when this occurs the two diseases are very difficult to distinguish from each other. However, some clinical symptoms and brain imaging findings suggest that vascular disease is playing a role in, if not completely explaining, a patient's cognitive impairment[246].*

Mild and slow vascular dementia symptoms creep into one's life. To complicate matters, just as there are several types of dementia, as Alzheimer's Society explains, there are also different vascular dementias:

"There are {several} types of vascular dementia. They differ in the {cause} and the part of the brain that {affected}," Alzheimer's Society said. "The different vascular dementia {types} have some symptoms in common, and some symptoms that differ. Their symptoms {progress} in different ways[247]."

How prevalent is Vascular dementia?

Vascular dementia accounts for almost twenty percent[248] of dementia cases and happens when damaged blood vessels cause bleeding of the brain.

Some sources suggest vascular dementia is the third most prevalent dementia, while others such as the National Institute on Aging and The Lancet Neurology[249] list vascular dementia as second behind Alzheimer's disease.

The actual number of vascular dementia and Lewy body dementia cases remains dubious because the available numbers remain estimations and dated. Doctors often misdiagnose both, and the estimated range could place either in second place.

Since this is not a horse race, I care not which is second or third. Both are prevalent and devastating dementias, so the focus should be on developing accurate and cheap testing, efficient and affordable prevention, and a reversible and permanent cure for all early stage dementia.

What Causes Vascular Dementia?

Blocked or diminished blood flow denies the brain oxygen and nutrients, killing brain cells, causing vascular dementia.

Vascular dementia-related blood flow issues occur in three primary ways and distinguish each subtype.

Narrowed small blood vessels in the brain cause Binswanger Disease, while a series of mini-strokes cause multi-infarct dementia, and stroke-induced blood clots cause post-stroke dementia[250].

Before we examine risk factors, let's probe each subtype's cause.

Vascular Dementia Types

This book focuses on two primary vascular-related dementias:

1. Cortical dementia
2. Binswanger Disease

While they are similar enough to classify as vascular dementia, they differ in their causes and how they destroy the mind.

Let's discuss cortical dementia first, which includes two subtypes: post-stroke dementia and multi-infarct dementia.

Chapter 16: CORTICAL VASCULAR DEMENTIA

Cortical vascular dementia comprises two subtypes:

1. Post-stroke dementia
2. Multi-infarct dementia

We discuss post-stroke dementia before addressing multi-infarct dementia. Strokes cause both vascular dementia subtypes, but not the same way.

Post-stroke dementia

Also called post-stroke cognitive impairment, post-stroke dementia occurs in about one/third of stroke patients[251].

According to the Barrow Neurological Institute Stroke Symposium, stroke survivors risk post-stroke dementia (vascular dementia) because of four overlying elements[252]:

1. Strokes cause significant brain tissue damage
2. Age-related cognitive decline risk
3. Amyloidopathy (pre-existing fragilities)
4. Comorbid vascular risks

According to a Stanford University Medicine study released in *Brain Journal of Neurology*, inflammatory activity two days following strokes show chances of severe cognitive loss a year later[253].

Marion Buckwalter, MD, Ph.D., associate professor of neurology and neurosurgery, Stanford University Medical School, explained the significance.

"Being able to identify early on," said Buckwalter, "patients who are at risk for dementia is a first step toward figuring out how to treat those at-risk patients[254]."

Post-Stroke Dementia Causes

While post-stroke dementia causes remain ambiguous, according to an *Annals of Translational Medicine* study, "the neuroanatomical lesions caused by the stroke on strategic areas such as the hippocampus and the white matter lesions (WMLs), the cerebral micro-bleeds (CMBs) due to the small cerebrovascular diseases and the mixed AD with stroke, alone or in combination, contribute to the pathogenesis of post-stroke cognitive impairment[255]."

Strokes prevent blood flow to the brain, denying it vital oxygen and nutrients.

Let's discuss the other cortical vascular dementia subtype, multi-infarct dementia.

Post-Stroke dementia symptoms

Post-stroke dementia follows a singular stroke. Depending on the severity of the stroke and brain area affected, post-stroke dementia causes the following symptoms.

- Agitation
- Attention-deficit
- Behavioral changes
- Calculation decline
- Cannot follow instructions
- Confusion
- Delusions
- Executive function decline (planning and organizing difficulties)
- Getting lost in familiar places
- Hallucinations
- Judgment decline
- Moodiness
- Short-term memory loss
- Wandering

How about multi-infarct dementia?

Multi-Infarct Dementia

Multi-infarct dementia strikes most victims between ages 60 and 75 and a higher percentage of men than women[256]. Most people have high blood pressure who develop multi-infarct dementia.

My Health Alberta describes multi-infarct dementia[257]:

> *Multi-infarct dementia is a loss of memory, thinking, judgment, or other mental skills caused by a series of strokes. A stroke occurs when {something blocks} blood flow to a part of the brain for a short time. If blood flow stops for too long, brain cells die. This leads to a loss of {motor and perhaps cognitive} skills.*

Because strokes are involved, brain damage is permanent. Healthy lifestyle changes are the best way to reduce stroke and vascular dementia risks.

Multi-Infarct Dementia Causes

A series of strokes blocks blood flow to the brain, damaging tissue, causing multi-infarct dementia[258].

The strokes causing multi-infarct dementia are mild, most transient ischemic attacks or ischemic strokes, but grow more intense, even fatal as the disease advances.

According to a University of Exeter review of 48 studies, including 3.2 million people, they found strokes double dementia risk. Lead author Dr. Ilianna Lourida reported the findings.

"We found that a history of stroke increases dementia risk by around 70%, and recent strokes more than doubled the risk," said Lourida. "Given how common both stroke and dementia are, this strong link is an important finding. Improvements in stroke prevention and post-stroke care may, therefore, play a key role in dementia prevention[259]."

The large-scale study confirmed stroke's crucial link to dementia. "Around a third of dementia cases are {potentially} preventable, though this estimate does not {consider} the risk associated with stroke," said Lourida. "Our findings indicate that this figure could be even higher and reinforce the importance of protecting the blood supply to the brain when attempting to reduce the global burden of dementia[260]."

Multi-Infarct dementia symptoms

As the name implies, multi-infarct dementia results from multiple strokes. Multi-infarct dementia symptoms strike suddenly and include:

- Arm weakness
- Bladder problems
- Bowel control decline
- Dizziness
- Getting lost in familiar surroundings
- Leg weakness
- Money handling problems
- Shuffled steps
- Slurred speech
- Unusual crying
- Unusual laughing
- Wandering

Initial symptoms might be mild or asymptomatic, but the above list occurs once anti-infarct dementia blocks enough small blood vessels.

Chapter 17: SUBCORTICAL DEMENTIA/BINSWANGER DISEASE

Otto Binswanger[261] first described the medical condition in 1894, and Alois Alzheimer[262] coined the term and improved the definition in 1902. Still, the profession credits Dr. Olszewski in 1962 for advancing the criteria used today.

The medical profession also calls Binswanger disease:

- Binswanger encephalopathy
- Multi-infarct dementia, Binswanger type
- Subcortical arteriosclerotic encephalopathy (SAE)
- Subcortical ischemic vascular disease
- Vascular dementia, Binswanger type

Binswanger disease often occurs with Alzheimer's disease, called mixed dementia[263].

Defined by cerebrovascular lesions in the hemispheric white matter, Binswanger disease images help doctors diagnose the condition[264].

For years, the medical community has debated whether Binswanger disease is an individual disease or arteriosclerotic ischemic damage.

Science Direct explains the controversy[265]:

> *White matter microinfarcts with vasculopathy are common in patients with underlying hypertensive disease, and some pathologists maintain that Binswanger disease is nothing more than severe white matter damage due to hypoxia/ischemia. {It} is difficult to determine that a dementing syndrome is explained by an ischemic process in the absence of any other cause of dementia in this widely and quickly expanding field.*

Controversies come with the territory in the dementia research community, for each dementia classification resulted from a grueling process where setbacks rivaled breakthroughs before reaching consensus.

The Medical community lumped LATE, the newest dementia classification, with Alzheimer's until April 2019, when a National Institute of Health-sponsored international workgroup defined LATE's criteria.

Until we understand how many dementias exist and develop accurate cheap tests, prevent and cure cognitive-related dementia, the struggle continues.

Our knowledge grows each day, but have we reached a point where we know more than not? Answering the question is difficult because we have chipped at the mountain for decades, but it still stands tall and formidable.

One fact is obvious. Binswanger disease knowledge far exceeds Dr.

Binswanger's discovery in 1884, Dr. Alzheimer's refinement in 1902, Dr. Olszewski's considerable contribution in 1962, as researchers continue to expand our understanding today.

According to the International Psychogeriatric Association, "present with extensive white-matter lesions and multiple lacunae on neuroimaging. SIVD {Subcortical dementia is} a more homogenous subtype of vascular cognitive impairment and dementia[266]."

Binswanger disease causes

Atherosclerosis (artery thickening and narrowing) causes microscopic brain damage in the brain's subcortical area by cutting off blood flow and denying the brain necessary oxygen and nutrients, causing Binswanger disease[267].

Binswanger disease symptoms

Binswanger disease differs from the other two vascular dementias because artery blockage causes damage to the subcortical area.

Symptoms include:

- Irritable
- Attention-deficit
- Clumsiness
- Falling (unexplained)
- Forgetfulness
- Moody
- Personality changes
- Psychomotor slowness
- Short-term memory loss
- Unexplained urinary problems
- Unsteady gait

"Subcortical dementia is a clinical syndrome characterized by slowness of mental processing, forgetfulness, impaired cognition, apathy, and depression," said Dr. JL Cummings[268].

V. ALZHEIMER'S-RELATED DEMENTIAS

- Alzheimer's Disease
- Early onset Alzheimer's
- Limbic-predominant Age-related TDP-43 Encephalopathy (LATE)
- Posterior Cortical Atrophy
- New Alzheimer's drug

Chapter 18: WHAT IS ALZHEIMER'S DISEASE?

Alzheimer's is an "irreversible, progressive brain disorder," according to the National Institute on Aging[269], "that slowly destroys memory and thinking skills, and, eventually, the ability to carry out the simplest tasks."

Alzheimer's disease accounts for sixty to eighty percent of all dementia. Scientists don't know the exact numbers because doctors often misdiagnose the different dementias for each other. Adding to the confusion, Alzheimer's is often present with other types of dementias[270].

A minimum of twenty percent of people suffering from other forms of dementia also end up with Alzheimer's. It's one of the most prevalent, devastating, and cruel diseases of our day.

Who discovered Alzheimer's disease?

In 1906, Dr. Alois Alzheimer discovered Alzheimer's when studying the brain of a woman who suffered cognitive decline, erratic behavior, and a diminished ability to communicate in the years, leading to her death. Before Dr. Alzheimer's discovery, the medical world and families lumped Alzheimer's patients into the "crazy" or "lost their mind" category. Most of the world is only now learning what Dr. Alzheimer knew in 1906.

The disease blindsides the average family when it strikes a member.

As difficult as the disease remains today, one can only imagine the indignities and horrors victims suffered before Dr. Alzheimer's discovery.

Alzheimer's Canada explains the discovery.

> *Dr. Alois Alzheimer first identified the disease in 1906. He described the two hallmarks of the disease: 'plaques,' which are numerous tiny, dense deposits scattered throughout the brain that become toxic to brain cells at excessive levels, and 'tangles,' which interfere with vital processes, eventually choking off the living cells. When brain cells degenerate and die, the brain markedly shrinks in some regions*[271].

Dr. Alzheimer discovered entangled lumps of fiber, now called tau (neurofibrillary or tangles), and unusual clusters on the woman's brain since named amyloid plaques.

Other Alzheimer's definitions

Let's turn to some respected authorities and see how they define Alzheimer's. The Alzheimer's Association defines Alzheimer's:

> *Alzheimer's is a type of dementia that causes problems*

> *with memory, thinking, and behavior. Symptoms usually develop and get worse over time, becoming severe enough to interfere with daily tasks*[272].

Alzheimer's causes memory deficits and erratic behavior. While symptoms develop slowly, Alzheimer's becomes debilitating in later stages.

Let's review the Mayo Clinic's definition: [273]

> *Alzheimer's disease is a progressive disease that destroys memory and other important mental functions. At first, someone with Alzheimer's disease may notice mild confusion and difficulty remembering. Eventually, people with the disease may even forget important people in their lives and undergo dramatic personality changes.*

The Mayo Clinic affirms the Alzheimer's Association's definition.

UK Alzheimer's Society

Let's turn to the UK and review how the Alzheimer's Society defines Alzheimer's[274]:

> *Alzheimer's disease is the most common cause of dementia. The word dementia describes a set of symptoms that can include memory loss and difficulties with thinking, problem-solving, or language. These symptoms occur {from} {atrophy caused} by certain diseases, including Alzheimer's disease.*

The Alzheimer's Society confirms Alzheimer's disease causes memory loss and inhibits one's ability to communicate and solve problems.

Life becomes more complex every day as the disease progresses until becoming the new norm.

Alzheimer's disease attacks the brain and destroys one's personality, much as rampaging barbarians who pillage a village until it is no more.

Since there is no cure, there are only three things we can do regarding Alzheimer's:

1. Adopt a lifestyle to slow or prevent Alzheimer's.
2. Continue the search for a cure.
3. Ease the burden on victims and their loved ones.

In stage one, Alzheimer's shows no symptoms.

An Alzheimer's diagnosis shocks, but there is no time to waste. Now is the time to live like there might not be a tomorrow.

Besides preparing for the future, embrace the earlier stages of the disease and squeeze as much quality time as possible. This stage is the last ride of normalcy, so make the most of it.

Let's review Alzheimer's relationship with dementia.

What is Alzheimer's relationship to dementia?

Much like China is one country within Asia, Alzheimer's is one dementia. As China is the largest country within Asia, Alzheimer's is the most prevalent dementia.

The different dementias share many symptoms, often causing misdiagnosis.

Adding to the confusion, doctors cannot confirm it is Alzheimer's until one dies, and they perform an autopsy. We need tests to detect different dementias, including Alzheimer's.

Plaques, neurofibrillary Tangles, Communication Breakdown

When studying Alzheimer's, the terms *amyloid plaques, neurofibrillary tangles,* and *loss connection* appear because they are the markers of the disease. Let's examine each, starting with amyloid plaques.

Amyloid Plaques

Beta-amyloid is a single-molecule protein that forms plaque in the brain and clumps into amyloid. The toxic plaque grows and disrupts the synapses connecting the brain's neurons.

The amyloid plaques form in the brains of people who do not have Alzheimer's, but the clumps are smaller. Those with Alzheimer's have a higher concentration of plaque in the hippocampus area of the brain responsible for emotions, learning, and memory.

A team of Stanford and Harvard scientists investigated how beta-amyloid elevates the risk of Alzheimer's. Carla Shatz, Ph.D., professor of neurobiology and biology and senior author of the study, shared their results.

"Our discovery," said Shatz, "suggests that Alzheimer's disease {manifests} long before plaque formation becomes evident." Shatz also reported[275]:

> *Beta-amyloid begins life as a solitary molecule but {bunches} up – initially into small clusters that are still soluble and can travel freely in the brain, and finally into the plaques that are hallmarks of Alzheimer's. The study showed for the first time that in this clustered form, beta-amyloid can bind strongly to a receptor on nerve cells, setting in motion an intercellular process that erodes their synapses with other nerve cells.*

Such discoveries add one more layer to the challenge but get us a step closer to understanding what causes Alzheimer's, so we can find a cure. Science is conducting and analyzing tests to determine why amyloid plaques develop and how to prevent them from damaging neurons.

We next study neurofibrillary tangles.

Neurofibrillary tangles

What Dr. Alzheimer referred to as "tangled bundles of fiber," now called neurofibrillary tangles, are uncommon levels of the tau protein that form inside neurons.

Normal tau protein protects neurons, but abnormal or muted versions accumulate inside and kill neurons, causing Alzheimer's symptoms, including abnormal behavior, memory loss, inability to organize and plan.

Why are tangles and plaques a problem? Before we move on, let's examine how the brain functions and how the tangles and plaques cause issues.

Loss of connection

The plaques and tangles break the connections (synapses) between the brain's neurons (nerve cells). When this happens, the brain functions much like an electronic device with a short in the wiring. If the neurons are unconnected, the brain cannot send messages to other brain parts, muscles, and organs within the body[276].

Neurons

Close to 100 trillion branches connect about 100 billion nerve cells in the brain and nervous system in a neuron forest. This vast communication network allows the different brain parts to function and us to direct our body parts.

When the neurons cannot transmit messages, the affected parts of the brain and body break down, arms will not move unless the brain commands. The brain's neuron network travels from head to toe, controlling all body parts.

Alzheimer's attacks the hippocampus area of the brain, the part that stores and processes memory, but spreads to other areas of the brain as Alzheimer's develops.

A fatal disease that kills and has no cure is cruel because Alzheimer's moves in methodical steps to block the connection between neurons and removes one's memory, reasoning skills, thinking ability, recognition skills, and advanced-stages attacks motor skills organs.

Communication is a critical component of life, and much is going on behind the scenes; we remain oblivious. When Alzheimer's destroys the neurons' ability to communicate, everything that is us disappears.

Science is still probing to find what causes amyloid plaques and neurofibrillary tangles. Still, one group of scientists believe they have discovered a vaccination to block both the amyloid plaques and neurofibrillary tangles from growing.

University of Texas (UT) Southwestern Medical Center develop Alzheimer's vaccine

Unsuccessful until now, the researchers at the UT Southwestern Medical Center developed a vaccine to "arm the body to attack Alzheimer's plaques and tangles before they {shut} down the brain[277]."

Scientists have conducted extensive and successful tests on mice. While such tests on animals do not always work on humans, the results remain promising, and scientists push forward.

Director of the UT Southwestern Alzheimer's Disease Center, Dr. Roger Rosenbert, explained the potential breakthrough[278]:

> *The significance of these findings is that DNA Aβ42 trimer immunotherapy targets two major pathologies in AD – amyloid plaques and neurofibrillary tangles – in one vaccine without inducing inflammatory T-cell responses, which carry the danger of autoimmune inflammation, as found in a clinical trial using active Aβ42 peptide immunization in patients with AD {Alzheimer's}.*

Testing humans and getting FDA approval is a lengthy process, but we hope they soon develop vaccines to spare most people from Alzheimer's and other dementias.

At what age do Alzheimer's symptoms first occur?

There are two versions of Alzheimer's, young or early onset Alzheimer's and regular Alzheimer's, the former rare and genetic, the latter prevalent, and science suggests caused by nongenetic factors.

The primary difference between the two is early onset strikes younger people in their forties and fifties.

Young or Early Onset Alzheimer's

Young or early onset Alzheimer's attacks people in their forties and fifties[279]. The medical community estimates 200,000 Americans have early onset Alzheimer's[280].

Almost identical symptoms as typical Alzheimer's, early onset Alzheimer's hits people decades before the regular version strikes.

According to Johns Hopkins Medicine, most people with early onset Alzheimer's have the standard version, but a few hundred have Genetic (familial) Alzheimer's disease. Those with these rare genes experience symptoms as early as age thirty[281].

Regular Alzheimer's

There is a reason many refer to Alzheimer's as the "old folks disease." The first signs appear in a person's mid-sixties[282].

How many people have Alzheimer's disease?

This section will investigate how many people have Alzheimer's in the United States and worldwide. Officials believe the actual numbers are much higher.

We know the numbers are worse than we can verify because of inadequate health systems in the third world and difficulties diagnosing Alzheimer's (no accurate test) worldwide.

"Some people with the disease never receive a diagnosis," said officials at the National Institute on Aging. "Many others have dementia-related conditions, such as aspiration pneumonia, listed as the primary cause of death while the underlying cause, Alzheimer's, {goes unreported}[283]."

Despite the limited data, enough death certificates list Alzheimer's as a cause of death to make the disease the sixth leading killer in the United States.

Authorities compute the numbers from death certificates and scientific studies, which causes them to underestimate the total. You could add ten or twenty percent and perhaps reach a closer number, but we use the more conservative official numbers for this discussion.

First, we will focus on the United States numbers, then examine global numbers.

How many Alzheimer's cases are there in the United States?

With a new case every 65 seconds[284], 5.7 million Americans[285] live with Alzheimer's.

How many Americans die from Alzheimer's?

In 2014, the last time they updated their numbers, the CDC attributed 93,500 American deaths to Alzheimer's disease[286].

These are the latest numbers. When officials release more recent official figures, we will update this section. The updated numbers should be much higher as the number of people with Alzheimer's has continued to rise.

More Americans die from Alzheimer's than heart disease, breast cancer, and prostate cancer totaled[287].

We need a better system

Officials should enter death certificates into a national pool in the computer age. The entry should include cause of death, a copy of the birth certificate, and any related disease such as Alzheimer's, cancer, diabetes, or any other ailment that perhaps caused pneumonia or whatever listed cause of death on the certificates.

It seems everybody in the world has our information except those who need it to do good. A national computer network would provide instant updates on the causes of death and help achieve more accurate information.

Such a system would arm medical researchers with more accurate and updated information, doctors with more weapons to diagnose and treat diseases, and patients with a better chance of recovery.

Instead of trailing other industrial countries, the United States must develop a quality health care system the rest of the world wants to copy. The current disastrous American and global health systems of diagnosing, treating, and reporting are insufficient.

How many Alzheimer's cases are there in the world?

There is a new case of dementia every 3 seconds, with Alzheimer's representing the majority[288]. Authorities diagnose almost 10 million people each year, and 50 million live with the disease worldwide[289].

By 2050, experts predict the numbers will reach 12.7 million[290].

How many humans die each year from Alzheimer's?

Getting an exact number of Alzheimer's deaths in the United States is difficult because death certificates often list pneumonia or some associated disease as the cause of death. Worldwide, the job is impossible.

The World Alzheimer's Report 2018 illustrates the problem and calls every nation to step forward to meet the challenge:

> *Many countries have no diagnostic tools, no access to clinical trials and {few} specialized doctors and researchers. Where those are present they may not have the means to travel and to communicate their ideas. Yet, with the biggest increases in dementia occurring in LMICs, does this make sense? Shouldn't the governments of those countries try to contribute to research for the benefit of their populations rather than relying on other countries, such as the USA and the UK, to lead the way*[291]*?*

The suggestion is easier said than done in countries already struggling to keep their heads above water. The words seem somewhat harsh, considering how impoverished the poorest countries are, but as we will soon address, costs threaten to bury even the most prominent and wealthiest nations.

Every three seconds, somebody in the world gets Alzheimer's or one of the other dementias.

There are 50 million global cases of dementia. Because of misdiagnosis and reporting issues, this number is likely much higher.

How many people worldwide die from Alzheimer's?

Worldwide, dementia—Alzheimer's, representing 60 to 80 percent—is the fourth leading cause of death, totaling 2.38 million[292].

Dementia (Alzheimer's) kills more people than:

- Lower respiratory infections
- Neonatal deaths
- Diarrheal diseases
- Road incidents
- Liver disease
- Tuberculosis

- Kidney disease
- Digestive disease
- HIV/AIDS
- Suicide
- Malaria
- Homicide
- Nutritional deficiencies
- Meningitis
- Protein-energy malnutrition
- Drowning
- Maternal deaths
- Parkinson's disease
- Alcohol disorder
- Intestinal infectious diseases
- Drug disorder
- Hepatitis
- Fire
- Conflict
- Heat or cold-related deaths
- Terrorism
- Natural disasters

Alzheimer's and the dementias kill more people than every other disease except for cardiovascular disease, cancers, and respiratory disease.

While the official numbers are staggering, we know the total as Alzheimer's and dementia numbers are low.

To American and global government and medical officials

Beller Health calls on the governments and medical communities of the world to step to the plate and provide researchers instant, detailed information about the cause of death, other health conditions, and other invaluable health data.

There are privacy and legal issues to work through. Still, there is too much avoidable human death and suffering because researchers often estimate what medical records should make crystal clear.

Do it if privacy issues mean blackout names, addresses, and other personal information. The information people want to protect is unnecessary. Researchers need age, cause of death, medical history, notes of importance for medical research.

Help save and enhance lives by providing accurate information!

Does Alzheimer's Discriminate?

We investigated whether Alzheimer's discriminates against any groups. What we found is the disease discriminates against:

Elderly
The most significant Alzheimer's risk factor is age[293].

Females
Although the science is unclear, women represent two-thirds of Alzheimer's patients[294].

African Americans
African Americans are two to three times as likely, as whites to get Alzheimer's[295].

Diabetes and high blood sugar
Several studies suggest diabetes and high blood sugar elevates the risk of Alzheimer's[296].

Down syndrome
People with down syndrome have a 50-50 chance of getting Alzheimer's[297].

High blood pressure
Higher blood pressure increases the risk of Alzheimer's[298].

Inactive minds
Inactive minds increase the chance of Alzheimer's. The brain needs exercise, too[299].

Obesity
Being overweight raises Alzheimer's risk[300].

Physical inactivity
Physical inactivity is dangerous and elevates the risk of Alzheimer's[301].

Unhealthy diets
Nobody can do anything about being elderly, female, African American, or having Down syndrome. However, a healthier lifestyle will help us avoid obesity, idle minds, lack of exercise, diabetes, and high blood pressure. Besides the higher risks to other diseases, the Alzheimer's numbers should wake us all up to how important it is to feed and exercise our bodies and minds.

Of the list, two stand out and require closer examination: females and African Americans.

Do Women Have A Higher Risk Of Alzheimer's?

While Alzheimer's does not discriminate by race, the disease strikes older people and females in disproportionate numbers. The higher number of females is in part because they outlive males.

United States

The life expectancy in the United States ranks 53 out of 100 nations where such statistics exist. The average American male lives 76.99 years, and females 81.88 years[302].

United Kingdom

In the UK, Alzheimer's and other dementias kill more women than any single alternative cause of death[303]. Also, of all UK Alzheimer's and dementia cases, 61 percent are female, and only 39 percent are men[304].

Worldwide

Women are 2.5 times more likely than men to get Alzheimer's[305]. According to the World Health Organization, Alzheimer's is the fifth leading global cause of death for women[306].

Alzheimer's and dementias strike women harder than men in the US, the UK, and worldwide.

Let's review the numbers for African Americans.

Do African Americans Have A Higher Risk Of Alzheimer's?

United States

According to one analysis of dozens of studies, the researchers concluded African Americans are under-represented and more unwilling to participate[307].

This reluctance might result from historical abuses such as the Tuskegee experiments. Whatever the reason, scientists and researchers must earn this trust, and African Americans must take part in studies for science to figure out what causes the higher ratio of Alzheimer's among the African American population.

Victimized in the past by systematic bigotry, African Americans fear unfair treatment if diagnosed with Alzheimer's.

Let's review the UK and global numbers to determine if the trend is exclusive American.

United Kingdom

A group of researchers studied 2.5 million people. The study found black women were 25 percent more likely to suffer Alzheimer's or dementia than white women, and black men were 28 percent more likely than white men[308].

One of the leading authors, Dr. Tra My Pham, of UCL's Institute of Epidemiology and Health, explained their findings.

"What we found suggests that the rates of people receiving a diagnosis may be lower than the actual rates of dementia in certain groups, among black men," Pham said. "It {concerns} that black people appear to be more at risk of dementia but less likely to receive a timely diagnosis[309]."

Science does not know the exact cause for the higher rates, but Dr. Claudia Cooper offered insight into the study's lead author. "Our new findings may reflect, for example, that there are inequalities in the care people receive to prevent and treat illnesses associated with dementia," said Cooper. "Or perhaps GPs or patients' families are reluctant to name dementia in communities where more stigma {associates} with a dementia diagnosis[310]."

We see a similar pattern in the US and UK. Are these consistent with global trends? It is impossible to say, for we could not find any credible data. We hope new data will shed new light on the subject, which we add in the next annual edition.

We have learned that Alzheimer's and dementias attack all groups but strike women and black people harder than whites and Asians.

Based on known Alzheimer's risks, what combination would make the perfect Alzheimer's candidate?

Perfect Alzheimer's candidate

An overweight, 65-year-old African American female who does not exercise, eats unhealthily, has high blood pressure and diabetes, does not challenge her mind, and suffers from Down syndrome would be the perfect candidate for Alzheimer's. She would carry ten high-risk factors, four out of her control and six within.

Like everybody else, women and black people need to view the risk factors under their control. While a few elements are beyond our best efforts, every human must develop better habits for the components we govern. We must demand more from the authorities in funding impartial studies for accurate tests, cures, and better treatment for a disease that destroys the golden years for over a third of humans fortunate to make it to their sixties.

Next, we will review the financial costs of Alzheimer's.

How Much Does Alzheimer's Cost?

No thorough discussion about Alzheimer's can exclude financial costs. If we do not find a cure or cheaper, better treatment for this disease, it will bankrupt most countries by 2050. The individual and government costs are already reaching unbearable levels.

We will break the costs into four categories:

1. Individual
2. United States
3. Global
4. Volunteer caregivers

Although enormous, this section does not focus on human costs. While we emphasize the financial hardships, we are not implying the economic costs are more significant than the horror those carrying the disease must endear, nor the difficulties caregivers face.

Before discussing the national and global costs, let's review the individual costs, and the estimated financial hardship on voluntary caregivers.

Individual costs

Besides the human suffering by the patient and families, the costs for treating one person with Alzheimer's is a minimum of $424,000, and this does not include the family's lost wages[311].

Families around the world make tough decisions when one member suffers Alzheimer's/dementia. A stable middle-class family can fall through the cracks.

Profit motives and other factors price medical care for diseases like Alzheimer's out of the reach of most Americans and global citizens, who have modest incomes, bad or no health insurance

United States Costs

As a nation, Americans spent a minimum of $277 billion in 2018 and will surpass $1.1 trillion by 2050 unless we win the war against Alzheimer's and dementias[312].

The Alzheimer's Association reports:

This {2018 cost} is approximately 48 percent of the net value of Walmart sales in 2017 ($481.3 billion) and nine times the total revenue of McDonald's in 2016 ($24.6 billion).

The US 2022 dementia costs, including Alzheimer's, is $321 billion, straining Medicare and Medicaid, which cover $206 billion of the total.

When politicians talk about waste, they should be ashamed for not funding accurate testing and cure research for Alzheimer's. Americans suffer on the level of continuous long-term torture, and the costs are bankrupting families and our health care system, but politicians are MIA in an actual war.

What are the estimated world costs?

Global costs related to Alzheimer's and dementia surpass one trillion dollars and will double by 2030, if not before. Like the United States, international human and financial costs are overwhelming families and governments.

Please review the Alzheimer's/dementia global costs.

YEAR	GLOBAL ALZHEIMER'S CASES	COST
2018	50 million	$1 trillion
2050	152 million	$9.12 trillion

Journal of the Alzheimer's Association[313].

The reported United States and global numbers are low. As people age and become the largest living generation, these costs will become unbearable for the younger generations.

Alzheimer's and dementia destroy individuals, families, and countries. Preventing Alzheimer's and the other dementias should be in the top three priorities of every nation in the world.

Volunteer Caregivers

Alzheimer's is a 24/7 job in the later stages, and much of this burden falls on volunteer caregivers. Besides the horrors for Alzheimer's patients, volunteer caregivers suffer significant financial loss, depression, stress, often resulting in health issues.

Over 16.1 million Americans provide 18.4 billion hours of volunteer care worth $232 billion to people carrying Alzheimer's and the dementias[314].

As you can see, Americans devote an enormous amount of care to loved ones suffering from Alzheimer's. The figures only account for what it would cost to hire somebody to do the work of volunteers and do not include the enormous amount of lost wages.

Other than those with Alzheimer's, nobody carries a more significant burden than those who offer invaluable voluntary care.

We will next face one of Alzheimer's frustrating realities.

What Causes Alzheimer's?

Whatever causes Alzheimer's disease deserves a chapter, but science offers little but a hypothesis and preliminary tests on lab animals. Until they find a breakthrough, this chapter remains incomplete.

For decades, the world's top neurologists have failed to determine Alzheimer's exact cause. Not knowing the cause, all Alzheimer's drug trials fail.

Discovering the cause (s) should provide researchers the information they need to develop accurate tests for Alzheimer's like they do cardiovascular and other diseases. Researchers and the medical community uncovered several risk factors but no cause.

Section four probes the risks, providing clues about preventing or slowing the disease.

For now, that is the best science offers.

We hope researchers soon give us a reason to rewrite this chapter and describe the exact cause (s) of Alzheimer's disease. We debated whether to include this chapter and emphasize its importance. The elusive cause is essential to finding a cure. Therefore, this chapter remains incomplete.

Let's examine Alzheimer's subtypes.

Alzheimer's Subtypes

Complicating efforts to cure Alzheimer's, evidence shows there is not one Alzheimer's but a minimum of three.

Several researchers and neurologists pointed towards Alzheimer's variances for decades, arguing one size does not fit all cases. The argument picked up steam in 2015 after back-to-back studies confirmed what neurologists long observed.

A two-year study released in 2015 by UCLA built on smaller research and determined there is not one Alzheimer's but at least three versions. The study's lead author, Dr. Dale Bredesen, a UCLA professor of neurology and distinguished neurodegenerative disease researcher, led the team.

"Because the presentation varies from person to person, there has been suspicion for years that Alzheimer's represents more than one illness," said Bredesen. "When laboratory tests go beyond the usual tests, we find these three distinct subtypes[315]."

In 2020, we believed there are three Alzheimer's subtypes:

1. Typical Alzheimer's
2. Posterior Cortical Atrophy (pre-dominant posterior atrophy or Benson's syndrome or parietal-dominant atrophy)
3. LATE (Limbic-predominant age-related TDP-43) or Medial Temporal Atrophy

Every piece we find in the Alzheimer's and dementia puzzle reminds us how little we know overall. In part explaining why a cure remains beyond our reach, each subtype causes different symptoms and requires other remedies.

Most drug trials and research focus on Alzheimer's as a singular disorder, but the subtypes explain, in part, why all drug trials have ended in failure. There will not be one cure, but we might discover a cure for each by discovering the subtypes.

A breakthrough in treating cancer provided hope to those who suffer or treat Alzheimer's and dementia. When researchers sequenced tumor genomes and compared them to patients' genomes to develop a systematic and exact treatment plan, those interested in an Alzheimer's cure noticed. Dementia patients and doctors hoped modern medicine could do the same with Alzheimer's disease.

In Alzheimer's, however, there are no such tumor or biopsy markers as cancer. How did the UCLA team overcome this obstacle?

"So how do we get an idea about what is driving the process?" said Bredesen. "The approach we took was to use the underlying metabolic mechanisms of the disease process to guide the establishment of an extensive set of laboratory tests, such as fasting insulin, copper-to-zinc ratio, and dozens of others."

Researchers identify over 100 disorders leading to dementia. While we focus on the 19 causing 99% of dementia cases, the fact remains there are over 100 dementia subtypes. There might be a dozen or more subtypes when science figures out more of the Alzheimer's puzzle.

Three Alzheimer's Types

According to neurologist Dale Bredesen, Alzheimer's results from 1) inflammation, 2) inadequate nutrient levels, and 3) "other synapse-supporting molecules, and exposures." By separating Alzheimer's into three subtypes, Bredesen and other researchers found different treatments for each.

Instead of viewing amyloid plaque deposits as the cause, Bredesen and other neurologists consider the deposits the amyloid protein's effort to protect the brain from true Alzheimer's causes. These neurologists point to the wide range of Alzheimer's risk factors and diverse pathology to suggest there is not one Alzheimer's but four.

1. Inflammatory (Typical Alzheimer's)
2. Posterior Cortical Atrophy (Cortical)
3. Limbic-predominant age-related TDP-43 encephalopathy (LATE)

4. Early onset Alzheimer's disease

LATE represents many older people before misdiagnosed for typical Alzheimer's. Depending on how science proceeds, LATE is an Alzheimer's subtype or Alzheimer's-like dementia.

For this book, we link the subtypes to Alzheimer's and cover them as distinctive dementia types. While typical Alzheimer's remains the most prevalent, the other three subtypes combined total almost fifty percent of Alzheimer's cases, making each one of the twenty most widespread dementia types.

The United States Alzheimer's prevalence

6.25 million Americans have Alzheimer's[316], and the total will grow to 13.85 million[317] by 2060. To add weight to the number, the number of Americans who have Alzheimer's or dementia exceeds the population of 46 states[318].

The officials are negligent because they remain inactive against the most extraordinary human disaster and financial crisis facing Americans and the government.

YEAR	US ALZHEIMER'S CASES	COST
2018	5.8 million	$277 million
2050	13.8 million	$1.1 trillion

The numbers come from BrainTest[319], Forbes[320], Alzheimer's Impact Movement[321], Bright Focus Foundation[322], Alzheimer's Association's annual Alzheimer's Disease Facts and Figures[323].

Please note reality is much worse than the numbers above, which do not include the misdiagnosed cases or the Americans walking around with dementia and do not know.

According to the Bright Light Foundation, over 500,000 Americans die from Alzheimer's disease each year.

Alzheimer's and dementias are an epidemic and threaten the nation's financial security and American families. The dementia cost wipes out savings and bankrupt families, and the burden dumped on taxpayers is growing insurmountable. Like our health system, something must give on costs.

Global Alzheimer's

Across the globe, the disease is no less devastating. Many international medical authorities misdiagnose, under-treat, and under-report Alzheimer's. According to the Bright Focus Foundation, by 2050, there will be a minimum of 152 million people who have Alzheimer's or other dementia[324].

Over 50 million people fight Alzheimer's/dementia, exceeding the entire population of 187 of 195 countries[325] globally[326]. Since the numbers are under-reported, the situation is even worse. Yet there is no coordinated effort between governments to defeat this global epidemic.

Other than climate change, there is no more imminent threat to humans and the global financial market than Alzheimer's and the other dementias.

Alzheimer's disease (AD) symptoms

1. Delusions
2. Hallucinations
3. Memory Loss
4. Mood and Personality Changes
5. Poor Judgement
6. Losing things
7. Physical Abilities
8. Word Troubles
9. Time and Place issues
10. Visual Impairment

You need to pay attention to warning signs regarding Alzheimer's. Watch for dramatic changes to memory, habits, moods, and perceptions. If troubling patterns develop, act fast.

Alzheimer's disease symptoms manifest differently in each inflicted person. While the symptoms might show in a different order, most Alzheimer's patients develop the ten symptoms.

Chapter 19: EARLY-ONSET ALZHEIMER'S DISEASE (EOAD)

If Alzheimer's disease (AD) is a demon, early onset Alzheimer's disease (EOLD) is the devil.

This chapter defines EOLD and discusses how it differs from typical AD, its prevalence, and its causes.

How prevalent is early onset Alzheimer's (FAD)?

Many call early onset Alzheimer's a rare form of Alzheimer's, but this dementia series views it as a significant dementia category. Representing a minimum of 5-10% of Alzheimer's disease (AD), early onset familial Alzheimer's (FAD) adds up to a significant number of people.

5.5 million Americans live with Alzheimer's disease, meaning 200,000 to 550,000 live with FAD.

Genetic or sporadic EOAD

The medical profession categorizes early onset Alzheimer's disease (EOAD) as either familial (genetic) or sporadic. Most EOAD patients suffer the sporadic version.

Early onset familial Alzheimer's disease (EOFAD)

Researchers link three genes to early onset familial Alzheimer's disease (EOFAD).

- Presenilin 1 (PS1)
- Presenilin 2 (PS2)
- Amyloid precursor protein (APP)

Science links the above genes to chromosomes 1, 14, and 21.

The three genes account for only 1-3% of Alzheimer's cases but account for 60-70% of early onset Alzheimer's disease[327] (EOAD).

Thus, when we discuss EOAD, we usually mean the familial variety.

Early onset sporadic Alzheimer's disease

Sporadic means no genetic link. Accounting for most typical Alzheimer's, but only 30-40% of early onset Alzheimer's, the sporadic variety remains an uncompleted global-size puzzle with too many missing pieces.

While genes might still play a role in early onset sporadic Alzheimer's disease (AD), genetics only explains a minority of AD. Other factors such as toxins, oral infections, elevated blood sugar, and other known and unknown factors are more likely suspects.

Neurologist Dale Bredesen refers to these causes as 36 holes in the roof and argues you cannot repair a leaky roof by focusing on one hole. Rather than focus all energy on the amyloid plaque and tau tangles, Bredesen argues we must personalize a treatment plan for each patient.

By running tests to measure one's toxin exposure, blood sugar, and other contributors and treating each, Bredesen argues we can prevent or reverse Alzheimer's, and by extension, a model to treat other dementias.

How does Early-onset Alzheimer's Disease (EOAD) differ from Typical Alzheimer's Disease (AD)?

The name suggests the most critical difference. If we think of three generations of a family, Alzheimer's attacks the grandparent, and FAD the parent.

Symptoms do not show in most typical Alzheimer's patients until age 65 or older, but early onset manifests symptoms in people 30-60 years old. Early onset strikes people in their prime, while fighting to the top of their profession, in the thick of raising children, and otherwise fully engaged in life.

Many psychologists and neurologists warn the shock is much greater when young people receive an early onset Alzheimer's or another dementia diagnosis. Depression and anxiety often follow the first symptoms or diagnosis.

Age is an essential difference between early onset AD and typical AD but only one of several significant differences.

Early onset Alzheimer's also causes more myoclonus than typical AD. We discuss these sudden twitches more in the symptoms section.

What Causes Early-onset Familial Alzheimer's?

Whereas genetics plays a minor role in typical Alzheimer's and most dementias, there is a vital link in early onset Alzheimer's. Mutated genes in chromosomes 1, 14, and 21 cause early onset Alzheimer's.

As with most dementia, protein deposits and tangles are front and center.

Chromosome 21 mutations resemble typical Alzheimer's because of the resulting amyloid protein (APP) deposits. In contrast, mutated chromosome 1 causes presenilin 2, and chromosome 14 mutations cause presenilin 1 deposits.

Chromosome

Protective and snug in the nucleus, chromosomes carry DNA molecules and coils around histones (proteins) for nucleosomes[328].

Receiving one of each chromosome type from our mother and father, we are born with 46 chromosomes.

Chromosomes are autosomes or allosomes. Autosomes are chromosomes 1-22, while allosomes include chromosomes X and Y.

Females carry two copies of chromosome X, while males have one X and one Y. Thus, females carry chromosome XX and males XY.

Thousands of genes stretch from one end of a chromosome to the other, carrying necessary DNA instructions to construct the human body, vital proteins, and additional maintenance[329].

View the photo below to see the chromosome within the nucleus.

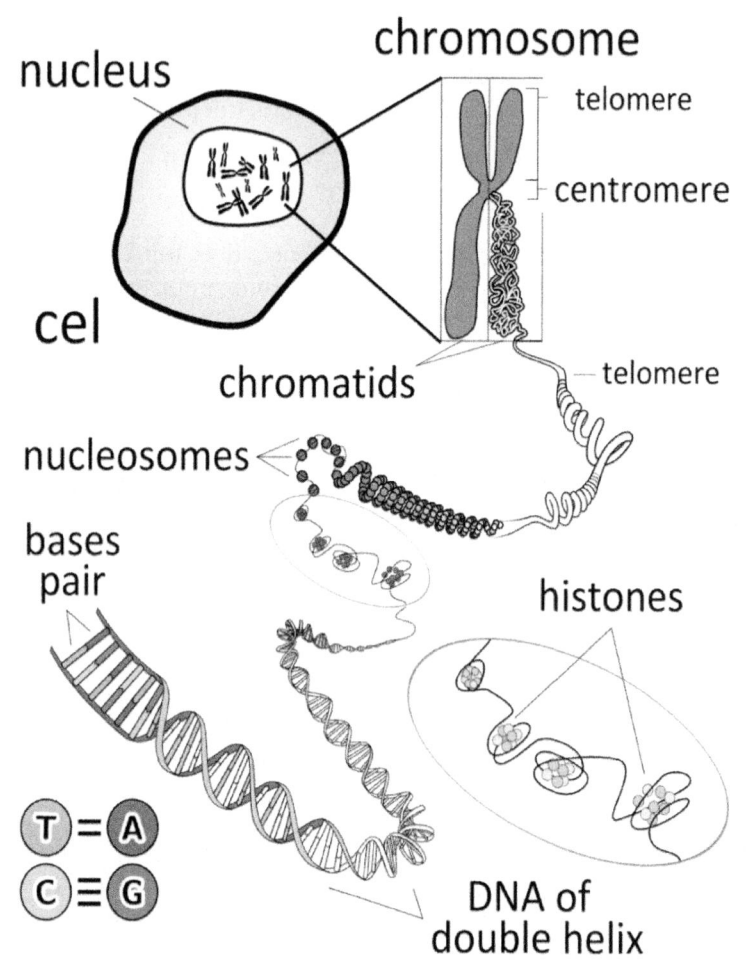

Chromosome err[330]

Let's discuss the three chromosomes linked to early onset Alzheimer's disease (EOAD), chromosomes 1, 14, and 21.

Chromosome 1

Including 249 billion DNA base pairs, the largest chromosome, chromosome 1, represents eight percent of DNA cells. Chromosome 1 contains 2,000 to 2,100 total genes[331].

Regarding early onset Alzheimer's disease (EOAD), we're interested in the

PSEN2 gene.

(PSEN2) Gene

The protein-coding gene, PSEN2, delivers code to produce APH-1, PEN-2, nicastrin, and presenilin proteins. We associate presenilin with EOAD.

Presenilin 2

A multiple gamma-secretase complex, presenilin 2 slices the amyloid precursor protein (APP) into smaller units called peptides[332]. Cleaving amyloid precursor protein (APP) prevents the accumulation associated with Alzheimer's.

Something occurs, causing presenilin 2 to malfunction, allowing Alzheimer's related protein accumulations.

Chromosome 14

Including 107 DNA building blocks, chromosome 14 represents up to 3.5 percent cellular DNA, a total of 800-900 genes. Each gene delivers instructions to produce essential proteins.

The chromosome gene connected to Alzheimer's is PSENI.

PSENI gene

The PSENI gene makes the Presenilin 1 protein, a proteolytic subunit of y-secretase.

Presenilin 1 Protein

Like presenilin 2, presenilin 1 breaks amyloid precursor protein (APP) into smaller pieces, preventing the buildup associated with AD.

For reasons little or unknown, presenilin 1 sometimes turns mutant and stops doing its job. Unmolested, APP clumps together and leads to Alzheimer's.

Chromosome 21

The smallest human chromosome and autosome, totaling 1.5% of cellular DNA, chromosome 21 contains 48 million nucleotides. Also called trisomy 21, there are 225 total genes in chromosome 21, compared to thousands in the larger chromosomes[333].

Linked to Down syndrome, Trisomy 21 also plays a prominent role in 50% of Down syndrome survivors getting Alzheimer's if they live to forty.

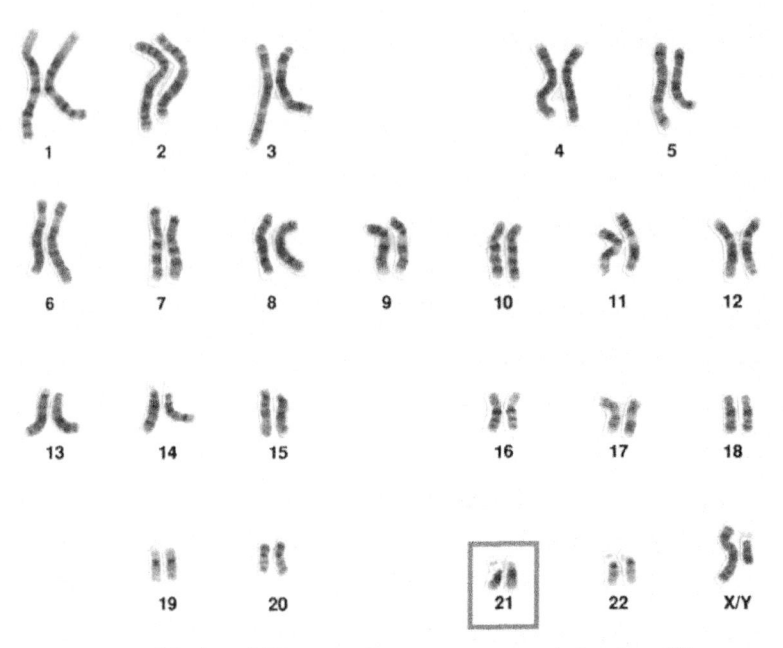

National Human Genome Research Institute[334]

Down syndrome with Alzheimer's disease is one of the 19 dementia types we cover in this series. Down syndrome represents one pathway to early onset Alzheimer's disease (EOAD).

Non (EOAD) Genetic Causes

Researchers link toxins, high blood pressure, and oral infections to Alzheimer's (early and typical versions).

Noted neurologist and researcher Dale Bredesen identified 35 mechanisms leading to Alzheimer's. Bredesen likens the mechanisms to 35 holes in the roof. For Bredesen, defeating Alzheimer's is a matter of identifying the underlying causes and treating each problem.

Bredesen's approach reversed Alzheimer's in dozens of patients by addressing the 35 underlying causes. To my knowledge, this is the only program to reverse AD.

Early onset Alzheimer's disease (EOAD) symptoms

The significant difference between early onset and typical Alzheimer's disease (EOAD) is the symptoms show before age 65 in the former. There are two types of early onset Alzheimer's; common and genetics. Most cases are common.

EOAD Early Symptoms

In the early stage, one might forget newly learned information or dates. A person asks for the same information, again and again. They experience difficulty solving fundamental problems, such as keeping track of bills or following a favorite recipe

Somebody with EOAD loses track of the date or time of year. EOAD symptoms cause some to forget where they are or how they got there. Depth perception or other vision problems often occur in the early stages.

Somebody with EOAD struggles to join conversations or find the right word. In the early stages, EOAD patients misplace things and cannot retrace steps to find the lost item.

EOAD patients suffer progressively poor judgment and changes in mood and personality. EOAD patients also suffer from mood swings and behavior issues. As a result, they withdraw from social and work situations.

AD symptoms

Let's discuss the more prevalent AD symptoms in greater detail.

Delusions

People with Alzheimer's suffer delusions that make them tough to manage. They view the world with paranoid eyes and often believe falsehoods that hurt those attempting to care for them[335].

People living with Alzheimer's suffering such delusions accuse family and caretakers of stealing their possessions.

Or falsely accuse the next-door neighbor of trying to take their husband or wife.

Or believe you are not who you claim.

People with Alzheimer's latch on to paranoia and fear and lash out at others. Nothing you say, not even presenting evidence to prove them wrong, will change their minds. The belief might be incredible to others, but Alzheimer's-related delusions are real to those suffering from them.

Loved ones must remember Alzheimer's is a severe disease, and those suffering possess little or no control over the symptoms. You cannot engage in arguments or otherwise chastise them for actions beyond their control.

The disease kills them in slow, methodical steps by robbing their ability to think, reason, perceive, and otherwise exercise the cognitive skills necessary for consistent everyday thinking. Alzheimer's patients accuse their loved ones and caregivers of awful things, but it's not their fault.

Please remember a demon called Alzheimer's attacked, and it is the disease driving the erratic and cruel behavior, not the person you've always known.

A point I shall risk repetition in this book: **Do not blame Alzheimer's patients for their behavior!**

Paranoia

One form of delusion, someone suffering paranoia associated with Alzheimer's, might believe others are out to get them. They suspect others of lying, cheating, cruelty, stealing, and other high crimes and misdemeanors.

They might look in the mirror and see a police car that is not there.

Or insist somebody is living in the attic.

11 things you should do or not do when a loved one suffers delusions and paranoia:

1. Ask the doctor if medications could cause the symptoms.
2. Check for cause and try to ease their concerns
3. Establish regular routines
4. Feed them well-balanced meals — lots of berries, nuts, vegetables, and wild-caught fish.
5. Keep answers short and elementary.
6. Reassure them.
7. Steer attention to something more positive.
8. Verify they are suffering a delusion and not something real.
9. Do not argue.
10. Do not convince.
11. Do not take offense.

The days of winning philosophical and other battles with the afflicted person are over! Do not argue, convince, or take offense at the delusional behavior.

Try to remember, as offensive and hurtful as it might be to you, what they experience is far more frightening. Cognitive abilities decline, and now they see unreal things that are their new reality. These fake things they experience are as real to them as they might be ridiculous to others.

When they believe somebody is living in the attic, or somebody is not who they claim to be, no matter how false, it could not be more real to those experiencing the delusions.

If they accuse you of being an imposter, it matters not if they have known you their entire life.

Be prepared! Once Alzheimer's strikes the sweetest person in the world, their meanest, most unreasonable moments test the most patient of souls and puncture those with the thickest skin.

Doctors treat symptoms with medication, which minimizes certain behavioral disorders. Some drugs are a godsend, while others only make the situation worse and risk too many dangerous side effects.

While people often confuse delusions and hallucinations, there are important differences, which we now examine.

Alzheimer's Hallucinations

Hallucinations differ from delusions. Whereas delusions cause believed falsehoods, people with Alzheimer's-related hallucinations experience sensory emotions that seem real to them. Alzheimer's patients not only see unreal people or things but smells odors, hear noises, hold conversations, taste, and feel to round out the hallucination[336].

Most hallucinations involve seeing and hearing people and things not there, although they might think they smell something they associate with evil or their childhood.

Hallucinations do not include mistaking something for something else, but believing something is there when it is not. In their heads, the imaginary things they see, touch, hear, smell, and taste are as real as their non-hallucinations.

What causes the hallucinations?

- Dim or flickering lighting could cause hallucinations in people with Alzheimer's.
- Broken routines, such as unfamiliar people and places, could explain the problem.
- Medication is a strong possibility, so report the issue and ask the doctor if medications could be the issue.
- Sundowning: a condition where those with Alzheimer's symptoms worsen later in the day.

The reasons for the hallucinations will differ for each person, but try the recommendations above and go from there.

The triggers differ for each person.

I suggest you keep a journal and make notes about each episode. Where did it take place? Who was present before and at the time of hallucination? List as much detail as possible. While it might not set off immediate alarms by itself, it might make more sense when you or the doctor reviews the journal.

The journal also can be therapeutic for loved ones and caregivers. Keeping a journal benefits the person with Alzheimer's and helps loved ones and caregivers focus on essential matters.

Do NOT use this journal to probe your emotional stress. Instead, use a personal diary or therapy to address your turmoil. Make the journal about the patient.

List as much as possible, including their eating and sleeping patterns, response to medication and therapy, delusion and hallucination triggers, physical mobility and balance, cognitive strengths and weaknesses, and anything you think is necessary.

What should you do when a loved one is suffering Alzheimer's-related hallucinations?

It is the same list as suggested for handling delusions:

- Ask the doctor if medications could cause the symptoms.
- Check for cause and try to ease their concern
- Do not argue
- Do not convince
- Check for a reason and try to ease their concerns
- Do not take offense
- Establish regular routines
- Feed them well-balanced meals — lots of nuts, berries, vegetables, and wild-caught fish
- Keep answers short and elementary
- Reassure them
- Steer attention to something more positive

Verify they are suffering a delusion and not something real.

Losing Things

We're not referring to misplacing keys or something minor that most do from time to time, but losing things and not knowing how. If somebody exhibits such symptoms, see a doctor[337].

The inability to retrace one's steps when one loses something is one of ten Alzheimer's symptoms that should ring the alarms. People with Alzheimer's often lose something, find themselves incapable of re-tracking their steps, and accuse somebody of stealing the missing item.

How does one know if it is typical aging issues or Alzheimer's?

The Cleveland Clinic explained usual memory issues, and something more serious like Alzheimer's[338]:

> ***Typical:*** *Misplacing things from time to time, such as a pair of glasses or the remote control.*
>
> ***When to seek help:*** *Putting things in unusual places, losing things, and being unable to go back over one's steps to*

find them again, accusing others of stealing.

Like other Alzheimer's symptoms in this book, one must remember it is the disease, not the person. No matter what kind of person they were before Alzheimer's, the disease takes over and removes the ability to process thought and regulate behavior.

Somebody with Alzheimer's might hide clothing in the freezer, the remote control in the dryer, keys in the oven, or any other imaginable misplacement.

By this point, a person should have already seen a doctor.

Once a doctor diagnoses Alzheimer's, it is crucial for caregivers and loved ones to lock up valuables, lock away or remove toxins, and minimize the number of places to hide things.

According to the National Institute on Aging, "there might be a logical reason for this behavior. For instance, the person may look for something specific, although he or she may not tell you what it is[339] causing difficulty for those suffering Alzheimer's and loved ones."

Next, let's look at perhaps the most immediate and prominent Alzheimer's symptom.

Memory loss

My shining days may be dimming, for sure, but life for me is not done/May God grant me peace, whatever those sunset days may bring.

— From a poem written by Alzheimer's patient John MacInnes

A retired executive and former pastor, MacInnes recognized he had a problem when he planned out a spectacular presentation as he had done many times on PowerPoint. But, the production did not go as dozens of others had before. "In mid-sentence, I had problems," MacInnes said, "I had a well-rehearsed script in front of me, but I couldn't get the words right, couldn't get them out. That kind of shook me up[340]."

From there, John struggled to multi-task, one of his former strengths. Next, he becomes disoriented while driving a few times. At age 80, John made an appointment, and his doctor diagnosed him with Alzheimer's. The early diagnosis allowed him to treat his symptoms and plan for the road ahead.

But how do we know it is not typical memory problems?

We all forget things. At our worst, we might even worry about ourselves. But it becomes more problematic if we can't remember recent events, names of people we know well, important dates we once processed, and need to make notes to reflect the most basic information[341].

Undiagnosed and unsuspected, in the early stages, amyloid plaque and neurofibrillary tangles are doing progressive damage to brain cells[342] (neurons or nerve cells).

Memory of smell

Losing the sense of smell is an early Alzheimer's memory symptom.

John Holger, MD, led a University Hospital Hamburg-Eppendorf review of 81 studies on Alzheimer's effect on smell memory.

Holger explained that Alzheimer's originates in the entorhinal cortex, the part of the brain that processes and communicates smell.

The meta-analysis of 81 studies confirmed people with Alzheimer's are "impaired on odor identification and recognition tasks," Holger said. "The impairment of smell recognition is of clinical importance, as patients often report malodorous sensations and changes in, e.g., the taste of foods leading to behavioral alterations. Consequences may range from increasing malnutrition to the development of delusions of poisoning that may trigger aggressive behavior[343]."

It is easy for loved ones to mistake the sudden changes in food tastes for somebody becoming difficult. They might one day turn hostile towards what had been their favorite meal.

"This feature of the neural network of smell memory," Holger said, "reflects the evolutionary pressure towards the secure recognition of 'bad' smells pointing to poisonous or rotten food that is pivotal for the survival of the organism."

Other memory loss symptoms

Memory loss is one of the first symptoms of Alzheimer's. We already covered the memory of smell and now will examine other examples of memory loss caused by Alzheimer's[344,345,346,347]:

- Can no longer manage medication
- Does not recognize familiar surroundings and gets lost while walking, driving, or shopping
- Does not remember anniversaries and birthdays
- Forgets recent events
- Forgets recent conversations
- Hides possessions such as keys or wallets in strange places such as the garage and forgetting
- Misses appointments
- Moodier than usual
- Repeats questions
- Struggles with routine tasks such as cooking or making coffee
- Word problems such as calling a cat a dog

Whatever one's standard memory before, it deteriorates once Alzheimer's symptoms show. If you or a loved one experiences any of the above or similar symptoms, see a competent doctor at once.

Whatever is causing the problem is serious; a diagnosis is vital, whether the problem is Alzheimer's or something else.

We next examine mood and personality changes somebody with Alzheimer's experiences.

Mood and personality changes

People with Alzheimer's struggle with moods and their personality changes. They're suspicious, anxious, often fearful, depressed, perplexed, insecure, and off-balance[348].

Verbal aggression

People with Alzheimer's struggle to process thoughts and lose their ability to screen what they say. If something pops in their mind, like a child, they say it without considering its appropriateness.

An agreeable person who never said an unkind word to anybody might become belligerent, contrary, insulting, arrogant, or otherwise aggressive. Somebody who once shied from confrontation might instigate conflict.

Physical aggression

The gentlest person in the world might go into a rage and destroy property or even threaten others. Some can no more control their physical aggression than screen what they say.

5 to 10 percent of those with Alzheimer's turn violent.

Michael Cohen described to CNN how his father went from a peaceful man to somebody his mother had to call 911 for breaking glass and threatening behavior. "It's like the 'Invasion of the Body Snatchers," said Cohen. "It looks like Dad, sounds like Dad, but it's not Dad[349]."

See your doctor and circle the family if you see signs in a loved one of violence. When somebody with Alzheimer's becomes aggressive, search for the cause and help defuse the situation.

Before we go to the next section, let's review the list of mood and personality changes associated with Alzheimer's.

List of mood changes caused by Alzheimer's

Mood changes related to Alzheimer's[350,351]:

- Aggression, anger, agitation
- Anxiety
- Calm and then upset without reason

- Delusions
- Emotionally unstable
- Fatigued all the time
- Hallucinations
- Happy, then sad for no reason
- More anxious than usual
- Physical outbursts
- Sleep issues
- Unprovoked anger and mood swings
- Unusual pacing

Chapter 20: LIMBIC-PREDOMINANT AGE-RELATED TDP-43 (LATE) OR MEDIAL TEMPORAL ATROPHY

We proposed a new name to increase recognition and research for this common cause of dementia, the symptoms of which mimic Alzheimer's dementia but [are] not caused by plaques and tangles (the buildup of beta amyloid proteins that Alzheimer's produces). Rather, LATE dementia is caused by deposits of a protein called TDP-43 in the brain.

—Julie Schneider[352]

Until 2019, doctors diagnosed Limbic-predominant age-related TDP-43 encephalopathy (LATE) as Alzheimer's. Lumping LATE, hippocampal sparing Alzheimer's, and posterior cortical atrophy explains, in part, why drug trials have failed.

In this book, we discuss the three as Alzheimer's subtypes. However, many view them as individual dementia types. Compared to posterior cortical atrophy, LATE closer mimics typical Alzheimer's.

LATE shares similar symptoms and pathology with Alzheimer's and frontotemporal dementia but differs from both.

Science uncovered not one vascular dementia but three, not one Lewy Body dementia but four primary subcategories, not one frontotemporal dementia but two primary subtypes, and not one Alzheimer's but four subtypes. As we learn more about the dementias, neurologists will add more subtypes to each primary dementia.

Is It Alzheimer's or LATE?

"Those of us who work in dementia have long been puzzled by our patients who have all the symptoms of Alzheimer's disease but whose brains do not contain the pathological features of the condition," said Howard. "We now know that these puzzling patients are probably suffering from LATE and not Alzheimer's disease and that LATE may be 'mimicking' Alzheimer's in about 20% of cases."

In the past couple of decades, several researchers pointed towards TDP-43 and suggested a new dementia type.

Researchers predict the medical profession misdiagnosed hundreds of thousands of people with LATE as Alzheimer's, meaning they administered the wrong medications and treatment[353].

Richard J. Hodes, MD, director of the National Institute on Aging (NIA), addresses a question many researchers and doctors ask.

"While we've {been} making advances in Alzheimer's disease research—such as new biomarker and genetic discoveries—we are {still} asking, 'When is Alzheimer's disease not Alzheimer's disease in older adults?" said Hodes. "The guidance provided in this report, including the definition of LATE, is a crucial step toward increasing awareness and advancing research for both this disease and Alzheimer's as well."

LATE "mimics" Alzheimer's, but they are different diseases.

Difference between LATE and Alzheimer's

Alzheimer's and LATE share similar symptoms but not pathologies.

Mutated TDP-43 protein unfolding causes LATE, whereas beta amyloid protein plaques and tau tangles cause Alzheimer's. Different protein deposits cause the two dementia types, and the deposits form in various brain regions[354].

The amyloid protein and neurofibrillary (tau) tangles attack the hippocampus and entorhinal cortex initially and later the cerebral cortex[355]. In the beginning, Alzheimer's attacks memory, while later causing declines in reasoning, language, and social behavior[356].

In LATE, the TDP-43 protein misfold in the amygdala brain region and causes episodic memory loss in the beginning. In the middle stages, the protein forms in the hippocampus and in the late stage in the middle frontal gyrus, which causes cognitive decline[357].

Diagnosing LATE is difficult because of it and Alzheimer's sharing symptoms. If not for the differing causes, they would be the same dementia. But, they have different protein sources and are contrasting dementias.

We have far to go in diagnosing Alzheimer's and LATE, especially the latter. Researchers and doctors have been developing the pathology for Alzheimer's for decades, whereas the science behind LATE's pathology remains in its infancy.

To know with certainty somebody has LATE, medical authorities must conduct an autopsy, the unfortunate reality for many dementias.

We need better, cheaper means to diagnose LATE, Alzheimer's, and the other dementias. Dr. Carol Routledge, Director of Research from Alzheimer's Research UK, addressed the problem.

"People are diagnosed with a specific form of dementia based on the symptoms they experience," said Routledge. "When the symptoms of diseases overlap, it is very difficult to {determine} the underlying cause[358]."

Although symptoms do not distinguish LATE from Alzheimer's, there are subtle hints. LATE develops slower than Alzheimer's disease[359], which provides contrast, if not clarity.

LATE History

The first pathological recognition of LATE occurred in a 1994 study when researchers discovered 13 patients had then-unnamed dementia. The study represents the first documented account of LATE.

Researchers and the medical community continued noticing, studying, and documenting LATE for 25 years until April 2019. The National Institute of Health sponsored an international group of researchers who named, classified and described the disease.

In a significant dementia breakthrough, the NIH-sponsored international neurologists' workshop confirmed, named, and explained LATE in the April 2019 edition of the journal *Brain*.

An international team including researchers from Australia, Austria, Japan, Sweden, United Kingdom, United States, and elsewhere named and defined a new dementia type, *LATE[360] (Limbic-predominant age-related TDP-43 encephalopathy)*.

Nina Silverberg[361], PhD., Director of the NIA Alzheimer's Disease Centers, and Richard J. Hodes[362], MD, director of the National Institute on Aging (NIA), co-chaired the workshop in Atlanta[363] in October 2018. They released their study's results in the journal *Brain* in April 2019, their findings making us reevaluate much of what we have believed about Alzheimer's and the broader category, dementia.

This book provides a basic overview of the new dementia category. We will expand the text as further studies on LATE emerge but use all available to describe a dementia condition previously classified as Alzheimer's.

While most dementia strikes seniors, some types strike infants as young as two. Study results show our topic, LATE (Limbic-predominant age-related TDP-43 encephalopathy), qualifies as a geriatrics medical condition.

One in four people over 85 has enough TDP-43 buildup to cause cognitive decline, deterioration of executive function, and memory loss[364].

Robert Howard, a professor of old age psychiatry at University College London, said, "Those of us who work in dementia have long been puzzled by our patients who have all the symptoms of Alzheimer's disease, but whose brains do not contain the pathological features of the condition. We now know that these puzzling patients are probably suffering from LATE and not Alzheimer's disease and that LATE may be 'mimicking' Alzheimer's in about 20% of cases."

This chapter defines the latest recognized dementia, LATE (Limbic-predominant age-related TDP-43 encephalopathy).

In the past couple of decades, several researchers pointed towards TDP-43 and suggested a new dementia type.

"People have, in their own separate bailiwicks, found different parts of the elephant," said Dr. Peter Nelson. "But this is the first place where everybody gets together and says, 'This is the whole elephant[365].'"

Dr. Nelson and dozens of research groups worldwide collaborated on the groundbreaking project over a decade.

Another member, Melissa Murray, PhD., molecular neurologist from the Mayo Clinic, explained their purpose: "develop diagnostic criteria for LATE, aiming both to stimulate research and to promote awareness of this pathway to dementia[366]."

Peter Nelson Explaining the Working Group's Purpose
Working Group Co-chair Peter Nelson[367] explained:

> 1. The consensus working group report on LATE was that – a distillation of what an international, multidisciplinary group could agree on.
>
> 2. The goal was not to produce a trendy new term. For me personally, a key goal was to have a diagnosis that could be made in a meaningful way. For example, at our center, we just signed out nine cases and four demonstrated what I can now call LATE-NC. It is not meaningful (or rather; it is needlessly puzzling) to patients, clinicians, or anybody else when different diagnosticians apply completely different terms and criteria for a **common phenomenon. The best e-mail I got in the past few days was from a respected colleague who wrote, "I already used LATE as a diagnosis today!"**
>
> 3. This was not a paper about FTD/FTLD. The commonalities and differences related to LATE-NC and FTLD-TDP were, naturally, a point of discussion among the group. Without getting down in the weeds, a consensus was not reached on that. Here are some differences that were agreed on and are highlighted in the paper: LATE-NC is ~100-fold more prevalent than FTLD-TDP (lifetime risk is 1:4 versus ~1:1000); LATE-NC [affects] people in a quantumly older age group; persons with FTLD-TDP [have] language and/or behavioral differences that have not been described in LATE; rather, persons with LATE-NC at autopsy [had] deficits in episodic memory. I, personally, would guess that those differences will be [correlated] with differences in the neuropathology, and other parameters, but time will tell. MAPT haplotypes make all sorts of tauopathies worse; doesn't make them all FTLD-Tau. Just as not all tauopathies are AD, not all TDP-43 proteinopathies are FLTD/ALS.
>
> 4. This is a massively underappreciated and understudied disease(s) – and yes, TDP-43 proteinopathy (with or without comorbid AD pathology) is strongly associated with cognitive impairment, although, for a gradually progressive disease

that affects >85-year-olds preferentially, a lot of persons die in a presumed preclinical state.

It is of course true that this is not the first word on age-related TDP-43 proteinopathy, nor, of course, the last. However, this is the first consensus group effort to address this topic, and it is hoped that this paper will help to move the field forward.

Peter Nelson wrote the above quote in Alzheimer's Forum in response to other researchers' thorough review and comments.

Several international researchers participated in the lively discussion. LATE is a hot topic within the medical community, and I applaud Nelson and his colleagues for their ground-shaking report.

Will future studies change some workgroup consensus findings, advance other theories, and address issues the workgroup did not?

I hope so!

Nelson and his distinguished colleagues did not present their findings as the final LATE or TDP-43 statement but instead provided a framework to address widespread dementia previously misdiagnosed. Again, well done!

Because of the work group's consensus, science can evolve and address the unanswered questions. The work group's findings provide researchers with a framework to study LATE as a separate disease from Alzheimer's.

Which brings us to an appropriate question: When is Alzheimer's not Alzheimer's?

Why is categorizing LATE important?

Bart De Strooper[368], molecular biologist, professor, University of London and the UK Dementia Research Institute, explained the importance of the new dementia category:

1. "It will refocus attention to TDB-43 physiology and stimulate work to find biomarkers for this pathology so we can make {the} more refined diagnosis.
2. It explains possibly to a certain extent why some trials in the Alzheimer's field failed: while they were curing the amyloid pathology, TDB-43 pathology just went on.
3. It will stimulate industry to find drugs against TDB-43 or related pathways[369]."

Not Frontotemporal Lobar Degeneration or Amyotrophic Dementia!

The TDP-43 protein also links to frontotemporal lobar generation and amyotrophic lateral sclerosis, but LATE is a separate medical condition.

How Prevalent is LATE?

According to Dr. Peter Nelson, LATE is a "disease that's 100 times more common than (ALS or FTLD), and nobody knows about it."

Nelson admits we do not yet know LATE's prevalence.

Data suggests LATE is rare for younger people but as prevalent as Alzheimer's in the oldest members of our species.

The international team of NIH-sponsored researchers who named and defined LATE estimate 20-50% above age 80 demonstrate the LATE-related TDP unfolding[370].

Can Somebody have LATE and Alzheimer's at the same time?

There is a dementia category called "mixed dementia" because multiple dementias are often present at once.

LATE and Alzheimer's are sometimes both present, and when this happens, the symptoms grow faster and are more devastating[371].

How does LATE change the way we view Alzheimer's?

Nina Silverberg, PhD., Director of the NIA Alzheimer's Disease Centers, explained why the LATE dementia classification affects our outlook on Alzheimer's and dementia.

"Recent research and clinical trials in Alzheimer's disease have taught us two things: First, not all the people we thought had Alzheimer's have it; second, it is very important to understand the other contributors to dementia," said Silverberg. "In the past, many people who enrolled in clinical trials likely were not positive for amyloid. Noting the trend in research implicating TDP-43 as a possible Alzheimer's mimic, a group of experts convened a workshop to provide a starting point for further research that will advance our understanding of another contributor to late life brain changes[372]."

Studies on the previously known dementias confirm how the medical community misdiagnosed other dementia types as Alzheimer's. The classification of LATE means the profession misdiagnosed all LATE cases for Alzheimer's in the past.

While this inflated Alzheimer's disease numbers (and led to more Alzheimer's research funds than other dementias), LATE patients have skewed Alzheimer's medication and treatment research outcomes.

Drug studies

The consensus group believes including LATE patients in Alzheimer's drug studies skewed the results.

"LATE probably responds to different treatments than AD, which might help explain why so many past Alzheimer's drugs have failed in clinical trials," said Dr. Peter Nelson. "Now that the scientific community {agrees} about LATE, further research into the 'how' and 'why' can help us develop disease-specific drugs that target the right patients[373]."

The consensus team recommends removing LATE patients from Alzheimer's drug trials and encourages independent studies for each dementia.

Learning what is not Alzheimer's helps pinpoint real treatment options. Drugs to treat Alzheimer's proteins might not work on LATE and, as Dr. Nelson suggested, explain why so many Alzheimer's drug trials fail.

LATE symptoms

LATE is the least documented and arguably the most difficult to research of the twenty dementias we cover. For decades, the newest classified dementia has been the mysterious "Alzheimer's" mystifying neurologists.

We need more studies to expand our knowledge of limbic-predominant age-related TDP-43 encephalopathy (LATE) symptoms. I cannot overemphasize the importance because to diagnose LATE, doctors must do so based on symptoms.

Neurologists and studies confirm LATE symptoms include:

- Episodic memory loss (usually the earliest sign)
- Emotional issues
- Behavioral issues
- Cognitive problems (not immediate, but later)
- Semantic memory loss (in the last stage, severe)

Limbic-predominant age-related TDP-43 encephalopathy (LATE) causes episodic memory problems early. Other early stage symptoms include emotional and behavioral issues.

The middle stage brings cognitive decline, often striking executive attention skills first.

Last stage LATE causes a wide range of memory and cognitive decline issues, rendering patients helpless. Pneumonia, respiratory infections, or injuries from falls are the most likely cause of death for LATE patients.

This section, like others, will probably change somewhat once more science develops for Limbic-predominant age-related TDP-43 encephalopathy (LATE).

Chapter 21: POSTERIOR CORTICAL ATROPHY

Also called Benson's disease, posterior cortical atrophy is an Alzheimer's variant. Although once lumped in with typical Alzheimer's, posterior cortical atrophy diverges in attacking the brain.

According to NIH, posterior cortical atrophy "is a neurodegenerative syndrome {characterized} by a progressive decline in visuospatial, visuoperceptual, literacy, and praxis skills. The progressive neurodegeneration affecting parietal, occipital, and occipito-temporal cortices which underlies PCA is {because of} Alzheimer's disease (AD) in {most} patients[374]."

Clinical imaging may or may not show atrophy for posterior cortical atrophy patients, complicating studies and diagnosis.

The UCSF Weil Institute for Neurosciences Memory and Aging Center defines posterior cortical atrophy.

> *Posterior cortical atrophy (PCA), also called Benson's syndrome, is a rare, visual variant of Alzheimer's disease. It affects areas in the back of the brain responsible for spatial perception, complex visual processing, spelling, and calculation[375].*

While rare compared to typical Alzheimer's, posterior cortical atrophy is more prevalent than several among the twenty most prevalent dementias.

How prevalent is posterior cortical atrophy?

PCA accounts for up to 5% of Alzheimer's cases, totaling over 200,000 per year, making it a significant dementia category.

What distinguishes posterior cortical atrophy from regular Alzheimer's?

Alzheimer's attacks short-term memory. In contrast, early posterior cortical atrophy symptoms are vision-related.

Posterior cortical atrophy Causes

Alzheimer's causes most cases, but Lewy body dementia, Creutzfeldt-Jakob disease, and other neurological disorders cause posterior cortical atrophy. People develop posterior cortical atrophy when the back of the brain shrinks, damaging the part responsible for visual processing and spatial perception[376].

Diagnosis

To make the correct diagnosis, neurologists and other medical professionals must know vital signs and symptoms, which help establish cause and improve the chances they order the proper tests and make the correct diagnosis.

Life expectancy

With no cure, posterior cortical atrophy life expectancy is 8-12 years from diagnosis[377].

Strikes younger than typical Alzheimer's

Posterior cortical atrophy distinguishes itself from Alzheimer's by striking people when they are younger. PCA symptoms manifest earlier than regular Alzheimer's. Whereas most people do not develop typical Alzheimer's until age 65 or older, posterior cortical atrophy symptoms often manifest in their fifties[378].

Posterior cortical atrophy strikes people younger because of specific damage to the back of the brain.

What causes posterior cortical atrophy?

While Alzheimer's is the most prominent path to posterior cortical atrophy, Lewy body dementia, or Creutzfeldt-Jakob disease, causes a minority of cases.

Posterior cortical atrophy symptoms

This chapter covers posterior cortical atrophy symptoms, then shows how they manifest through stages.

Posterior cortical atrophy distinguishes itself from Alzheimer's by striking people when they are younger. The contrast makes some ask: *How can Alzheimer's cause posterior cortical atrophy, but the latter's symptoms manifest quicker?*

Excellent question!

The answer lies in how long it takes somebody's Alzheimer's symptoms to show. Although Alzheimer's does not strike people younger than 65, the damage to the brain has taken place for decades.

Posterior cortical atrophy strikes people younger because of specific damage to the back of the brain. While symptoms might appear to be physical, the damage to the brain causes physical problems.

A trillion neurons in our brain communicate with each other and different parts of our body. Our bodies do what our brain instructs. We do not move our fingers, speak, walk, or otherwise engage our bodies without our brain sending the correct signal.

While Alzheimer's is the most prominent path to posterior cortical atrophy, other neurological causes include Lewy body dementia or Creutzfeldt-Jakob disease.

Posterior cortical atrophy symptoms

Posterior cortical atrophy symptoms manifest earlier than regular Alzheimer's. Whereas most people do not develop Alzheimer's until age 65 or older, posterior cortical atrophy symptoms often manifest in their fifties[379].

Although posterior cortical atrophy patients maintain writing and nonvisual language skills, they suffer other language and visual impairments.

The following are posterior cortical atrophy symptoms:

- Blurred vision

- Bright light & shiny surface sensitivity
- Coordinated movement impairment
- Depth perception difficulties
- Deteriorating calculation skills
- Double-vision
- Getting lost in familiar places
- Hallucinations
- Inability to see in low light
- Failure to recognize commonplace people and objects
- Reading difficulties (trouble following lines of text)
- Trouble pointing and reaching for objects
- Writing impairment

Scientists from the United States, the United Kingdom, Canada, Germany, the Netherlands, Belgium, Italy, France, Brazil, and Spain formed a workshop and established a consensus posterior cortical atrophy classification. They determined space perception and simultanagnosia are frequent symptoms. According to the workgroup, common symptoms include[380]:

- Object perception deficit
- Constructional dyspraxia
- Environmental agnosia
- Oculomotor apraxia
- Dressing apraxia
- Optic ataxia
- Alexia Left/right disorientation
- Anterograde memory deficit
- Acalculia Limb apraxia
- Prosopagnosia Agraphia
- Visual field defect
- Disoriented to time and place
- Impaired insight
- Verbal fluency agnosia
- Finger agnosia

We next focus on the less prevalent dementias.

VI. OTHER DEMENTIAS

This section covers seven less prevalent dementias.
- Amyotrophic lateral sclerosis
- Creutzfeldt-Jakob disease
- Wernick-Korsakoff syndrome
- Huntington's disease
- Normal pressure hydrocephalus
- Corticobasal syndrome
- Chronic traumatic encephalopathy

Chapter 22: AMYOTROPHIC LATERAL SCLEROSIS

Also called Lou Gehrig's disease, amyotrophic lateral sclerosis (ALS) is a motor neuron disease.

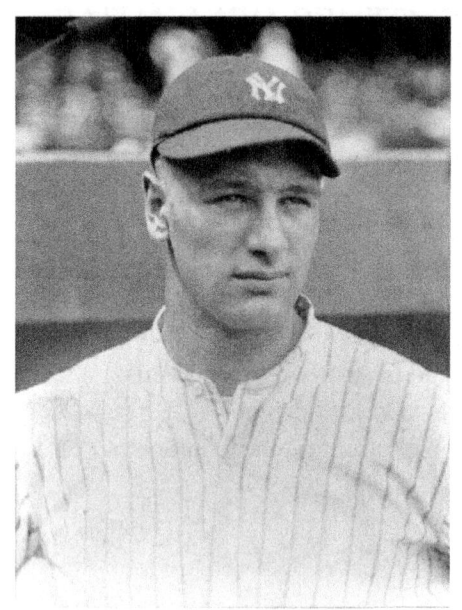

Lou Gehrig

Lou Gehrig was a baseball giant. He won almost every baseball award handed out while playing, including the most valuable player and six World Series Championships. The Baseball Writers Association of America voted him the most extraordinary first basemen to play the game.

He also became the face of amyotrophic lateral sclerosis (ALS).

One of the most famous people with ALS was a member of the science community. Stephen Hawking suffered ALS and defied the odds, surviving for 55 years after diagnosis. Hawking showed us two things: the symptoms in human terms and how one can still accomplish the remarkable. Most ALS sufferers do not experience the fulfilling life Stephen built, but each should create their version of greatness.

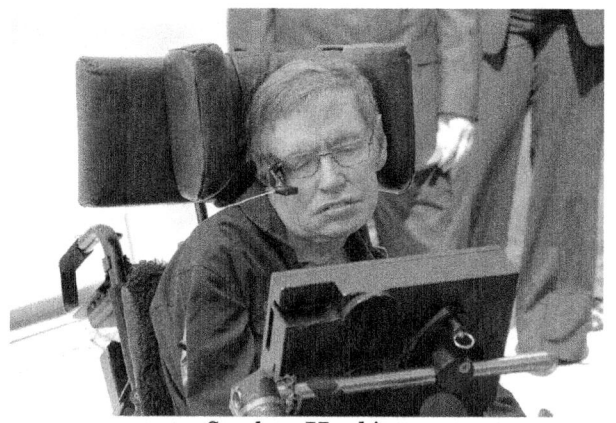

Stephen Hawking

ALS destroys motor neurons responsible for communication between the brain and voluntary muscles throughout the body. Incurable, ALS causes walking, talking, chewing, and other motor muscle-related problems[381].

Let's view an image diagramming ALS pathology and mechanisms.

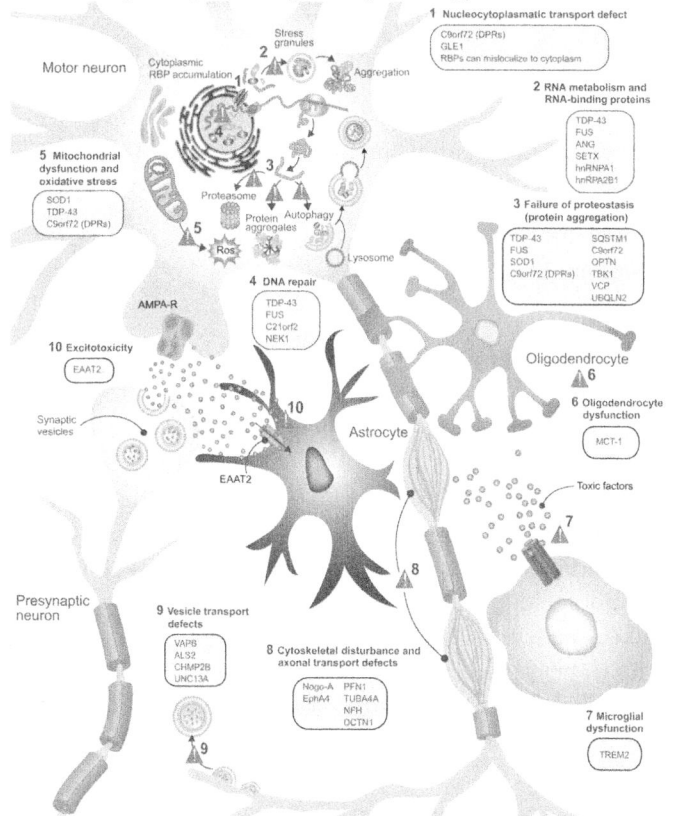

File: ALS Disease Pathology and Proposed Disease Mechanisms.jpg[382]

The image shows the ALS points of interest, marked by the red triangles with the exclamation points.

There are two types of ALS.

- Sporadic ALS
- Familial ALS

Sporadic ALS

Medical authorities consider about 90% of ALS sporadic, meaning a parent did not pass a mutated gene associated with familial amyotrophic lateral sclerosis.

The Muscular Dystrophy Association points to potential risk causes[383]:

1. Glutamate toxicity
2. Immune system abnormalities
3. Mitochondrial dysfunction
4. Oxidative stress
5. Toxic exposure

Next, let's discuss familial ALS.

Familial ALS

Familial means multiple family members suffer ALS. There are four ALS genetic categories:

1. Autosomal
2. Dominant
3. Recessive
4. X-linked

Autosomal

Most familial ALS is autosomal, meaning the mutation occurs in chromosomes 1-22, not in X or Y.

Dominant

Dominant familial ALS implies a parent passed one mutant chromosome gene to a child. Dominant familial includes chromosomes 1-22 and, like autosomal, does not include X or Y. A child of somebody with an abnormal dominant familial gene has a 50% chance of also getting ALS.

Recessive

Recessive familial ALS means both cell copies in the chromosome are abnormal. While parents show no signs of ALS, both carry and pass one abnormal cell to their offspring.

X-linked

X-linked ALS occurs when a parent passes a mutant cell in the X chromosome to a child. The abnormal cell can come from either a woman's two X or a man's one X chromosome.

What causes ALS?

The C9orf72 gene accounts for 25-40%, while Sod1 accounts for another 12-20% ALS.

There are three other genes responsible for the remaining ALS cases; TARDP, FUS, and VCP. X-linked inheritance and autosomal recessive patterns link to some incidents, but autosomal dominant explains most ALS cases[384].

The most common sporadic and familial ALS cause, C9orf72, instructs protein development in neurons in the brain's cerebral cortex and the spinal cord.

Crucial for sending and receiving motor neuron signals, researchers believe C9orf72 is essential in developing RNA. C9orf72 includes six nucleotides (building blocks), two cytosines, four guanines (GGGGCC), a hexanucleotide repeat[385].

Mutated C9orf72 protein leads to RNA foci accumulation. Toxic C9orf72 RNA sequesters RNA-binding proteins, damaging, then killing neurons[386].

Normal SOD1 protein destroys toxic radicals within cells. Instead of performing the toxic cleanup, rogue SOD1 unbinds zinc ions and intramolecular disulfide, causing the ALS-related fibrillar aggregates[387].

Less frequent ALS-associated genes include FUS, KIF5A, UBQLN2, and TDP43.

ALS prevalence

According to the ALS Association, a minimum of 16,000 Americans live with ALS, but Medscape[388] and others estimate the number closer to 30,000.

While not as prevalent as the primary dementias, an American gets ALS every 90 minutes, totaling 15 new cases per day and 5,000 each year[389].

ALS Global Prevalence

A minimum of 450,000 people worldwide has ALS[390].

Western Countries

In another indictment of the western diet and lifestyle, let's compare ALS prevalence worldwide to western countries. One out of 50,000 people worldwide get ALS, but one out of 20,000 in Western countries.

Eating a healthier diet, exercising more, sleeping 7-8 hours per night, better oral hygiene, limiting exposure to toxins, and other lifestyle changes are central in any legitimate effort to prevent or slow ALS or dementia.

Who gets ALS?

ALS strikes most people between 55 and 75 years old[391], men more significantly than women, especially in the non-familial version. Up to 93% of ALS patients in the United States are white, and 60% are male[392]. The reasons remain unclear, although the racial risk is striking.

Because of greater toxic exposure and unknown factors, soldiers and military veterans are twice as likely as nonveterans to get ALS[393].

Non-genetic reasons cause up to 90% of ALS.

Amyotrophic lateral sclerosis symptoms

Like strokes, initial amyotrophic lateral sclerosis (ALS) often focuses on one side of the body.

According to Stanford Medical School:

> *The first sign of ALS is often {a} weakness in one leg, one hand, the face, or the tongue. The weakness slowly spreads to both arms and both legs. This happens because as the motor neurons slowly die, they stop {signaling} the muscles. So the muscles {have nothing} telling them to move. Over time, with no signals from the motor neurons telling the muscles to move, the muscles get weaker and smaller[394].*

The initial motor issues in the face, tongue, hand, or leg might cause them to feel heavy. Beginning symptoms might produce minor weakness, but the atrophy kills motor neurons responsible for communicating signals from the brain to the tongue, face, hand, or leg.

ALS symptoms

- Ankle feebleness
- Atypical yawning
- Behavior or personality changes
- Cognitive decline
- Falling
- Feet fragility
- Hand weakness
- Leg weakness
- Slurred speech
- Stumbling
- Struggles with daily tasks
- Swallowing issues
- Twitching (Arms, shoulders, and tongue)
- Unnatural crying
- Unusual laughing
- Walking trouble

ALS symptoms sources: NORD[395], Mayo Clinic[396], Orphanet Journal of Rare Diseases[397], ALS Worldwide[398], Harvard Medical School[399]

Chapter 23: CHRONIC TRAUMATIC ENCEPHALOPATHY (CTE)

Although perhaps they should, most dementia conversations do not begin with the cause. However, our chronic traumatic encephalopathy (CTE) starts with the direct cause, traumatic heady injuries. Head injuries are complex, as the CDC story below illustrates:

> *In 1988, {a powerful boat struck} Dr. J.M.Z. – a 44-year-old marriage and family counselor – while kayaking and knocked unconscious for a short time. {The} hospital emergency department briefly examined and {said} he had suffered a "concussion" and {was} sent home an hour later without other treatment. Despite symptoms including headache, fatigue, and memory loss, he returned to his counseling practice. His clients noticed his memory and concentration problems, and he had to close his practice in six months. His health insurance company raised his premium rates until he could no longer afford coverage. His wife divorced him. His applications for Social Security disability income were denied over two years, and for six months, he had to live in a van. Finally, he received some Social Security benefits. Years later, he learned about and enrolled in a new college program designed for people with brain injuries. He developed ways of partially compensating for his continuing memory and concentration difficulties and re-opened a part-time counseling practice that provides minimal income. Appropriate follow-up from a State TBI registry might have led him to helpful programs earlier.*

The CDC tells the story above, illustrating the potential consequences of traumatic brain injuries.

Chronic traumatic encephalopathy (CTE) results from repetitive brain trauma. The leading cause of death in the United States for children and young adults, about 1.5 million Americans, suffer a traumatic brain injury each year. Of the 1.5 million, 50,000 die, up to 90,000 result in long-term disability, and 230,000 severe enough for hospitalization, but the people survive[400].

Worldwide, authorities estimate 69 million people suffer a traumatic brain injury each year[401].

High-risk chronic traumatic brain injury (CTE) candidates

- Athletes
- Soldiers
- Workers (in fields with frequent brain injuries)
- Newborns to four-years-old
- Young adults (age 15-24 the peak age)
- Males age one to 100 (males traditionally engage in more dangerous activities)

Anybody who suffers multiple head injuries risks chronic traumatic encephalopathy down the road.

Athletes rarely suffer chronic traumatic encephalopathy while still playing but strikes later once they've retired from sports. Same with soldiers, who are usually veterans by the time CTE symptoms develop.

In the United States, most jobs where most repeated head injuries occur require hard hats, such as construction sites. Such measures prevent serious injuries, but head injuries still occur at alarming rates. A hard hat does little good when one falls or gets knocked off the roof of even a one-story building.

Newborns are helpless and dependent, awkward and curious, and their heads not fully developed.

Young adults, primarily aged 14-24, create and engage in more voluntary dangerous activity than any other age group. They feel invincible, command an endless energy source, adrenaline addicted, and pursue any avenue with the potential for dopamine release. The comment is not an insult to young adults, for humanity needs youthful energy, alternative perspectives, and the greatness youth produces. But the never-ending quest to outdo the previous generation and each other also comes at a price. One is a disproportionate share of traumatic brain injuries.

Males suffer a higher percentage of head injuries. Traditionally, through occupation and recreation, mandatory and voluntary, males take far more risks than women.

Chronic traumatic encephalopathy (CTE)

Most dementia types take years or decades doing the underlying damage leading to dementia symptoms and hold with chronic traumatic encephalopathy.

One of the earlier studies (Corsellis, Brierley, et al., 1959) described CTE as progressive neurodegeneration resulting from hyperphosphorylated tau (p-tau) forming neurofibrillary tangles[402].

A brain autopsy study[403] (Corsellis, Bruton, et al., 1973) on boxing brains confirmed the 1959 (Corsellis, Brierley, et al.) study's results.

Anybody who suffered traumatic brain injuries (concussions), especially repetitive concussions, carries a higher risk for chronic traumatic encephalopathy (CTE) down the road. According to the Mayo Clinic, a person who suffers one concussion is likely to suffer another[404].

Brain autopsy on former National Football League (NFL) stars proves the relationship between concussions earlier and dementia later in life. One such autopsy study of a former NFL player by the University of Pittsburg (Omalu, DeKosky, et al., 2005). Omalu and the team reported their results:

> *Autopsy {confirmed} coronary atherosclerotic disease with dilated cardiomyopathy. The brain demonstrated no cortical atrophy, cortical contusion, hemorrhage, or infarcts. The substantia nigra revealed mild pallor with [a] mild dropout of pigmented neurons. There was mild neuronal dropout in the frontal, parietal, and temporal neocortex. Chronic traumatic encephalopathy was evident with many diffuse amyloid plaques {and} sparse neurofibrillary tangles and tau-positive neuritic threads in neocortical areas. There were no neurofibrillary tangles or neuropil threads in the hippocampus or entorhinal cortex. Lewy bodies were absent. The apolipoprotein E genotype was E3/E3[405].*

The description provides additional evidence for clinical diagnosis findings, confirming two or more CTE symptoms.

The combination of past traumatic brain injuries and two or more CTE symptoms point towards CTE.

Chronic traumatic encephalopathy (CTE) variations

An American study (Stern, Daneshvar, et al., 2013) concluded CTE clinical presentations[406].

- Behavioral and psychiatric
- Cognitive
- Motor

Behavioral and psychiatric CTE

Cognitive issues do not develop first in this variation, but aggression, apathy, delusions, depression, impulsiveness, and suicidal tendencies.

Cognitive CTE

Cognitive CTE causes a wide range of cognitive issues.

- Attention trouble

- Concentration decline
- Executive function deterioration
- Language deficits
- Memory problems
- Visuospatial decline

Motor CTE

Motor CTE causes ataxia, dysarthria, Parkinsonism-like tremors, and spasticity.

When diagnosed with traumatic encephalopathy (CTE) life prognosis, what age are most patients?

While dementia has a reputation for striking the elderly, the first CTE symptoms occur in most patients' twenties or thirties.

Chronic traumatic encephalopathy (CTE) prevalence

Considered the most extensive study of chronic traumatic encephalopathy to date, Mayo Clinic researchers (Bieniek, Blessing, et al., 2019) found almost 6% of the population suffers from CTE[407]. Bieniek told *Medscape Medical News*: "While [the] frequency of this disorder is not as high in amateur athletes compared to professional athletes, CTE pathology — of various levels of severity — is (present) in small, yet significant, number of cases[408]."

Chronic traumatic encephalopathy (CTE) symptoms

Up to this point, we described chronic traumatic encephalopathy and the responsible traumatic brain injuries. In most cases where past traumatic brain injuries lead to chronic traumatic encephalopathy (CTE), the symptoms do not appear for years or decades following the last brain injury.

Years or decades down the road, chronic traumatic encephalopathy (CTE) manifests some variety of the following symptoms:

- Apathy
- Cognitive impairment
- Depression
- Emotionally unstable
- Executive skills decline (including trouble planning and completing tasks)
- Impulsiveness
- Memory (short-term memory loss)
- Substance abuse

- Suicidal

Physicians should monitor traumatic brain injury patients and watch for any combination of listed symptoms. You should look for any of the above signs on every office visit, not for a few months or a year, but years or decades, however long they live and remain under your care. Once somebody experiences a head injury, they remain at high risk for chronic traumatic encephalopathy (CTE) for the rest of their life.

Suicidal

Evidence shows a higher risk of suicidal thoughts and actions by CTE patients than in general.

Brain Injury Research Institute, West Virginia University (Omalu, Bailes, et al., 2010) found a significant link between CTE and suicide[409].

University of Pittsburgh Medical Center researchers (Maroon, Winkelman, et al., 2015) performed a systematic review of confirmed CTE cases between 1954 and 2013. Maroon and team found an 11.7% suicide rate and 17.5% accidental death rate among CTE patients, compared to 1.5% and 4.8%, respectively, in the general population[410].

Closing traumatic head injury thoughts

Ideally, the physician watched for the symptoms after monitoring the patient for years or decades following past traumatic brain injuries.

Traumatic brain injury history + two or more CTE symptoms = chronic traumatic encephalopathy (CTE).

We need better programs to teach young people and others the potential long-term dangers of head injuries. Seeing men in their fifties come out of retirement to box professionally or other athletes continue to play after suffering multiple concussions makes me cringe. So do American football pickup games without helmets, states without motorcycle and bicycle helmet laws, and other examples suggest that society does not take head injuries seriously.

I call on the medical community to lead the charge, for it will not be coaches, CEOs, or anybody who benefits from the recklessness. Larger global health organizations must ring the alarm regarding traumatic head injuries.

Chapter 24: CORTICOBASAL SYNDROME (CBS)

Another FTD disorder, the first official report of corticobasal syndrome (CBS), was in 1967 when Jean J. Rebeiz and colleagues documented three patients with slow, clumsy movements that grew progressively worse[411].

Rebeiz and others continued to study the mysterious disorder for two more decades before WR Gibb and colleagues developed the name to corticobasal degeneration and provided an abbreviation (CBD) for a second distinction[412].

Also called CBS attacks the brain's frontal and temporal lobes.

To help form an image of CBS, the Baylor College of Medicine describes CBS as "a Parkinsonism-plus syndrome.

Atypical parkinsonism, corticobasal syndrome (CBS), attacks the brain's cerebral cortical and basal ganglia regions, responsible for motor movement. CBS causes problems with balance, muscle control, memory, and speech[413].

Although CBS shares some Parkinson's symptoms, they are two different disorders. Besides contrasting symptoms, CBS does not respond to treatment as Parkinson's.

According to the Journal of Neuropsychiatry[414]:

> *CBD is a neurodegenerative dementia with abnormal movements and focal behavioral manifestations. The clinical diagnosis is difficult to make in the absence of pathological findings. Functional imaging studies may be very helpful in demonstrating asymmetrical abnormalities in frontoparietal regions, basal ganglia, and thalamus contralateral to clinical symptoms, particularly in the early stages.*

What is the difference between corticobasal syndrome (CBS) and corticobasal degeneration (CBD)?

One glaring difference between CBS and CBD is their sometimes divergent pathologies. A specific tauopathy leads to corticobasal degeneration (CBD), but Alzheimer's sometimes explains corticobasal syndrome (CBS).

CBS prevalence

According to NORD, CBS attacks five of every 100,000 people[415].

Who gets CBS?

Most studies suggest that CBS assaults men and women in nearly equal numbers, although a few show women are at a slightly higher risk.

Although documented cases of corticobasal syndrome striking people as young as 28 exist, CBS strikes people aged 50-70 most of the time.

CBS life expectancy

From the time symptoms manifest, the average life expectancy is eight years. However, some do not make it for eight years, and others have survived up to 17 years.

What causes CBS?

Like many dementias, scientists remain baffled about what causes corticobasal syndrome (CBS).

We know tau protein buildup is associated with some CBS patients, while others exhibit the amyloid protein associated with Alzheimer's. However, we do not understand why the protein turns rogue[416].

If this story sounds familiar, it's the same old song with several dementias.

We have not developed a cure for CBS, Alzheimer's, and other dementias because we go about it wrong. Drug studies focus on reducing dementia-related protein deposits, but this is the equivalent of chopping a weed above the surface and does not treat the underlying problem.

In part, it might also explain why each drug trial costs billions of dollars.

Corticobasal syndrome (CBS) Symptoms

Often misdiagnosed for Parkinson's disease, corticobasal syndrome causes a wide range of symptoms affecting speech and language, memory and cognitive skills, movement, and motor skills.

This chapter outlines corticobasal syndrome symptoms and then discusses more in the stages section.

Corticobasal syndrome symptoms list

- Acalculia
- Akinesia
- Alien limb phenomenon
- Apraxia
- Bradykinesia
- Dystonia
- Visuospatial disorder

The list shows corticobasal syndrome attacking motor and cognitive skills. Before moving on, let's discuss each symptom.

Acalculia

Perhaps the rarest connection to corticobasal syndrome, acalculia attacks the part of the brain responsible for mathematics[417]. A person who skillfully handles math and develops acalculia might struggle with basic addition, subtraction, multiplication, and division.

Akinesia

People refer to CBS as atypical Parkinsonism because both disorders cause akinesia. When somebody has akinesia, they cannot make something move.

Somebody suffering from akinesia cannot move muscles voluntarily[418]. For instance, akinesia prevents the arms from swinging back and forth, usually without thought. Akinesia also causes other movement problems.

Damaged neurons cannot signal the muscles and nerves to move. Akinesia causes immeasurable frustration for CBS, Parkinson's, stroke, and other neurological disorders.

Alien limb phenomenon

The opposite of akinesia, alien limb phenomenon, causes involuntary movement. Also known as Dr. Strangelove's syndrome, alien limb phenomenon is a crucial CBS diagnosis factor[419].

Patients often feel separated from their limbs, and the movements cause significant stress.

Apraxia

Apraxia is the opposite of the alien limb phenomenon. A person experiencing apraxia cannot perform learned movements[420]. Aware of what they want to do, the brain no longer follows their commands.

Prominent in Corticobasal syndrome (CBS) is limb apraxia, which causes limited use or paralysis in an arm, hand, or leg.

The American Speech-Language-Hearing Association describes limb apraxia: "A disorder of motor planning in the absence of impaired muscle control that affects voluntary positioning and sequencing of muscle movements of the limbs[421]."

Stroke patients also suffer apraxia, which is why neurologists sometimes misdiagnose corticobasal syndrome for stroke.

Bradykinesia

Brain damage causes bradykinesia, a disorder causing slow movement.

Bradykinesia resembles akinesia, but they are not synonymous. The *Journal of Neurology* explains the difference:

> *Bradykinesia describes the slowness of a performed movement, whereas akinesia refers to a poverty of spontaneous movement (e.g., in facial expression) or associated movement (e.g., arm swing during walking).*

> *Other manifestations of akinesia are freezing, and the prolonged {time} to initiate a movement[422].*

Bradykinesia makes a person feel as if they are moving in slow motion. Whatever their normal speed, most movements are slow. Somebody suffering from bradykinesia struggles to tap their finger, tap a foot, or move palms up and down at any speed[423].

Dystonia

Dystonia causes uncontrollable muscle contractions in certain parts or the entire body.

According to the Dystonia Medical Research Foundation: "Dystonia can affect any region of the body including the eyelids, face, jaw, neck, vocal cords, torso, limbs, hands, and feet. Depending on the region of the body affected, dystonia may look quite different from person to person[424]." Dystonia Medical warns dystonia causes enormous anxiety and severe depression.

The American Association of Neurological Surgeons explains dystonia's complexity.

> *Dystonia is a very complex, highly variable neurological movement disorder characterized by involuntary muscle contractions. Two hundred fifty thousand people in the United States have dystonia, making it the third most common movement disorder behind essential tremor and Parkinson's disease[425].*

Parkinson's-like symptoms such as dystonia are why most consider corticobasal syndrome a Parkinsonism-plus disorder.

Visuospatial Disorder

Our visuospatial network helps create our unique vantage point.

Normal visual-spatial processing establishes our presence or place in the world compared to the space, objects, animals, and people around us.

Visuospatial disorder destroys the ability to make sense of objects, animals, and people surrounding us. Somebody suffering from a visuospatial disorder cannot find things a few feet away, including the bathroom or familiar objects[426].

The problem is not the eyes, which might be perfect, but our brain's ability to process, establish, and maintain our place in the world.

Visuospatial disorders make it difficult or impossible for one to determine distance. The breakdowns cause mass confusion and make it difficult for somebody to find something feet away from stairs (not recommended for somebody suffering from a visuospatial disorder) or the bathroom.

A severe visuospatial disorder places a person in a perpetual state of disorientation.

Chapter 25: CREUTZFELDT-JAKOB DISEASE

A rare but fatal degenerative brain disorder, Creutzfeldt-Jakob disease, is a common transmissible spongiform encephalopathy. A prion disease, Creutzfeldt-Jakob disease, causes holes in the brain until it resembles a sponge.

CJD

The National Institute of Neurological Disorders and Strokes (NINDS) describes Creutzfeldt-Jakob disease (CJD) as a "rare, degenerative, invariably fatal brain disorder[427]."

Mad cow's disease for humans

Creutzfeldt-Jakob disease is the mad cow's disease for humans, as Science Daily compares it to "Bovine Spongiform Encephalopathy (BSE) in cows and Chronic Wasting Disease in deer[428]."

100% Fatal

If a mad cow's disease for humans frightens, it should. The Centers for Disease Control and Prevention warns Creutzfeldt-Jakob disease is "always fatal[429]."

The National Institute of Neurological Disorders and Stroke reports Creutzfeldt-Jakob disease kills most victims within a year[430].

Creutzfeldt-Jakob (CJD) categories

According to NINDS, there are four categories of Creutzfeldt-Jakob disease (CJD), each deadly and representing a different pathology.

Only ten to fifteen percent of CJD is hereditary, and one percent is acquired, usually through contaminated surgical instruments. Most Creutzfeldt Jakob disease is sporadic, meaning no known genetic connection.

CJD Categories

- Sporadic Creutzfeldt-Jakob disease
- Familial Creutzfeldt-Jakob disease
- Variant Creutzfeldt-Jakob disease
- Iatrogenic Creutzfeldt-Jakob disease

Let's discuss each before advancing to the symptoms section. While similar, each diverges from the other, reaching the symptoms through different paths.

Think of apples at the supermarket. While all apples, one variety green, another red, one sweet, another tart. All four are different yet part of the same fruit family.

Like the apples, the four Creutzfeldt-Jakob disease (CJD) subtypes both resemble and differ.

Sporadic Creutzfeldt-Jakob disease (sCJD)

The most prominent prion disorder, sporadic Creutzfeldt-Jakob (sCJD) disease, accounts for 85% or more of Creutzfeldt-Jakob disease (CJD). According to the *American Academy of Neurology*, CJD develops in most patients in their sixties and often kills within months[431].
The UCSF Weill Institute for Neurosciences describes sCJD:

> *The cause of "classic" or "sporadic" CJD is unknown, which means it occurs in people {with no} known risk factors or gene mutations. Typical symptoms include imbalance and incoordination, memory loss and impaired thinking, and psychiatric symptoms such as anxiety or depression. Once the symptoms do appear, CJD progresses [quickly] and is usually fatal within a few months of symptom onset. sCJD typically affects people in their 60s and is rarely seen in people younger than 40 years old. Sporadic CJD is the most common form*[432].

Science works to uncover the exact cause but knows more about risk factors. When studying neurological disorders, I prioritize discovering lifestyle changes reducing dementia risks. While too many things in life remain beyond our control, for dementia risk factors, we control many.

Hereditary (Familial) Creutzfeldt-Jakob disease (hCJD)

Accounting for 10-15 percent of Creutzfeldt-Jakob disease, hereditary CJD strikes people younger than the other two subtypes, and symptoms develop slower. Hereditary CJD results when parents pass the mutant genes to their children.

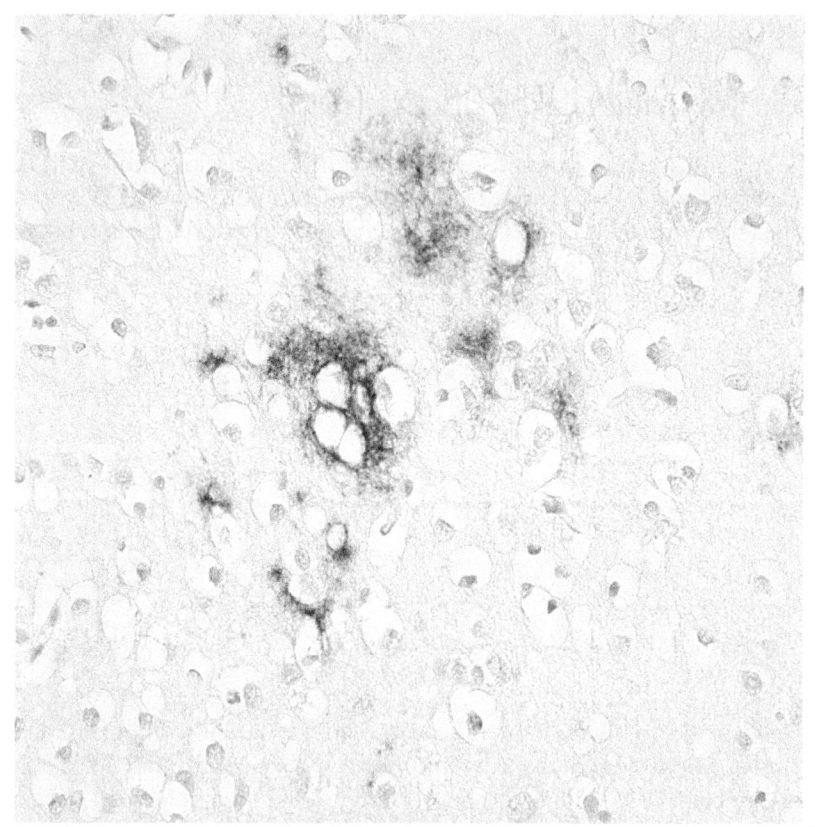

Prion_protein_immunostaining_(purple)_and_spongiform_change_in_the_brain_of_a_pa tient_with_Creutzfeldt-Jakob_Disease[433]

Iatrogenic Creutzfeldt-Jakob disease (iCJD)

Iatrogenic Creutzfeldt-Jakob disease is a reminder caring for sick people comes with many risks for surgeons, nurses, and medical officials.

Also called acquired CJD, iatrogenic Creutzfeldt-Jakob disease accounts for only one percent of the total Creutzfeldt-Jakob cases. The surgeon and team risk getting acquired CJD from surgical instruments and blood from surgery on CJD patients. Acquired CJD strikes people in their sixties and develops fast, killing within six months.

The first reported iCJD case in 1974 involved a patient who got iCJD from an infected corpse during a corneal transplant. Growth hormones and dura mater grafts account for most cases.

Medscape reports the reminder of iCJD cases results from "neurosurgical instrument contamination, corneal grafts, gonadotrophic hormone, and secondary infection with variant CJD transmitted by transfusion of blood products[434].

Iatrogenic Creutzfeldt-Jakob disease (iCJD) is rare and, in most cases, avoidable. Medical authorities have done an outstanding job recognizing the source(s) of the problem and adopting the safety features to all but eliminate this CJD subtype.

Educating surgeons, surgical teams, and other medical officials worldwide remain paramount in preventing iCJD. I applaud neurosurgeons and others who recognized and located the iCJD problem and the continued efforts within the profession to avoid the avoidable. Well done!

Variant Creutzfeldt-Jakob Disease (vCJD)

People (primarily Europeans) get this variation of Creutzfeldt-Jakob disease from eating contaminated beef.

According to the Centers for Disease Control and Prevention (CDC), "There is now strong scientific evidence that the agent responsible for the outbreak of prion disease in cows, bovine spongiform encephalopathy (BSE or 'mad cow' disease), is the same agent responsible for the outbreak of vCJD in humans[435]."

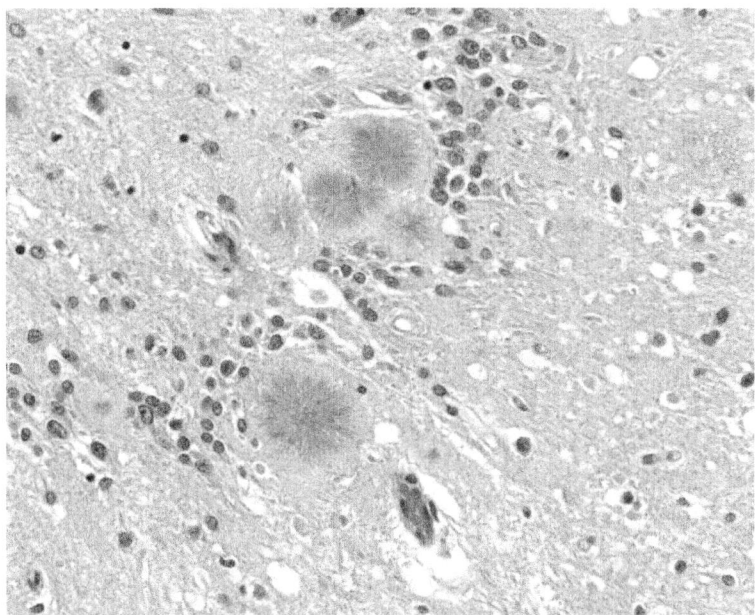

Variant_Creutzfeldt-Jakob_disease_(vCJD),_typical_amyloid_plaques[436]

Bovine Spongiform Encephalopathy (BSE)

Most of us remember the scare when the British first reported bovine spongiform encephalopathy in 1996 and immediately became known as mad cow disease.

vCJD

Natural Health Service warns there is an incubation period of ten years or more before vCJD manifests[437].

vCJD Strikes Them Younger

Variant Creutzfeldt-Jakob disease (vCJD) attacks people much younger than other CJD variants. According to the University of Rochester Medical Center, vCJD strikes people when they are an average of 28 years old[438].

Almost Wiped Out

Medical authorities learned from early variant Creutzfeldt-Jakob disease (vCJD) cases and nearly wiped out this variant since. However, several cases could still linger because of the long incubation period.

Creutzfeldt-Jakob disease (CJD) symptoms

The symptoms manifest, and how quickly they develop depends on the Creutzfeldt-Jakob disease subtype. The symptoms fall into two categories: neurological and psychological.

CJD symptoms

Psychological Symptoms

Early psychological symptoms include:

- Anxiety
- Depression (can be severe)
- Despair (acute)
- Insomnia
- Irritability
- Isolation (withdraws from family, friends, etc.)

Unlike other dementias where the early symptoms are mild, Creutzfeldt-Jakob disease develops severe symptoms from the beginning. Let's review early neurological symptoms.

Neurological symptoms

Early neurological symptoms include:

- Balance and coordination decline

- Body numbness
- Dizziness
- Slurred speech
- Vision decline (including double vision and hallucinations)

The combination of neurological and psychological symptoms strike and grow progressively worse.

Chapter 26: HUNTINGTON'S DISEASE (HD)

The most prevalent neurodegenerative malady is Huntington's disease (HD). Huntington's disease is also called Chronic Progressive Chorea, Degenerative Chorea, HD, Hereditary Chorea, Hereditary Chronic Progressive Chorea, Huntington's Chorea, VEOHD, Very Early Onset Huntington's Disease, and Woody Guthrie's disease. HD is a fatal genetic disorder that kills brain cells.

Like myotonic muscular dystrophy, Huntington's is an autosomal dominant inheritance disorder and poses the same threat to females and males[439].

If one has a genetic link to dementia, including everybody with Huntington's disease, it is a death sentence. A genetic link to any devastating illness is frightening.

I must stress not everybody who has a parent with Huntington's will get the disease. "Each child of an affected parent has a 50/50 chance of getting the mutant gene," according to John Hopkins Medical, "and therefore has a 50% chance of inheriting the disease."

Not inheriting the disease also breaks the Huntington's disease cycle, for a child who did not inherit the genetic mutation cannot pass it along to their children.

The US Library of Medicine describes Huntington's disease[440] as a "progressive brain disorder that causes uncontrolled movements, emotional problems, and loss of thinking ability (cognition)."

The symptoms might sound like Parkinson's disease, but there are apparent differences for those familiar.

Whereas Parkinson's disease is an akinetic-rigid syndrome, Huntington's disease is a trinucleotide repeat disorder. To help distinguish between the diseases, we will define both.

Let's discuss akinetic-rigid syndrome to help distinguish Parkinson's from Huntington's disease.

Akinetic-rigid Syndrome

According to Oxford Medicine, akinetic-rigid syndrome produces "paucity and slowness of movement accompanied by muscle stiffness and resistance to passive movement. The akinetic-rigid syndrome is typical of idiopathic Parkinson's disease, often described as the syndrome of parkinsonism[441]."

Our focus is Huntington's disease, so let's shift the discussion to trinucleotide repeat disorders.

Trinucleotide Repeat Disorders

A trinucleotide repeat disorder repeats genes, toxifies cells, creates an imbalance, and lays the groundwork.

"When the cause of a disease {is} having too many copies of a certain nucleotide triplet in the DNA, the disease {is} trinucleotide repeat disorder. Today, there are 14 documented trinucleotide repeat disorders that affect human beings[442]."

Huntington's disease is one of the 14 documented trinucleotide repeat disorders. Huntington's disease repeats the codon CAG, which codes for glutamine, an amino acid.

Having discussed causes for Huntington's disease, akinetic rigid syndrome, and trinucleotide repeat disorders, let's investigate what age the symptoms manifest.

What Age Does Huntington's Disease Strike?

Unlike most dementias, Huntington's disease strikes people in their prime. Ages 30-50 is when most people find their footing, come into their own, refine their goals, and chase new dreams.

According to the Pathology Department at the University of Pittsburgh Medical Center, on average, Huntington's strikes manifest when somebody is age 40, but strikes people as young as four and as old as 84, and the average lifespan from there is 13 years[443].

Within the margin of error, The Alzheimer's Association supports the numbers. Huntington's disease "usually develops between ages 30 and 50," Alzheimer's Association[444] said, "but they can appear as early as age two or as late as 80."

Huntington's disease is one of the crueler dementias in two ways:

1. Unlike most dementias, genetics causes Huntington's disease.
2. The primary victims are not towards the end but in the prime of life.

As cruel as the typical Huntington's disease version, another is even more terrifying.

Juvenile Huntington's (JHD) Disease

Juvenile Huntington's disease (JHD) is when symptoms show under age twenty. Less common, juvenile Huntington's disease accounts for 5-10% of Huntington's disease (HD) cases[445].

Once Juvenile Huntington's symptoms manifest, the lifespan is under ten years, less than half the adult version[446].

Juvenile Huntington's disease symptoms include: "changes in personality, coordination, behavior, speech or ability to learn," according to the Huntington's Disease Society of America. "Physical changes include rigidity, leg stiffness, clumsiness, slowness of movement, tremors, or myoclonus."

Any disease robbing kids' childhood churns my stomach and reminds me how random life is. When dementias strike older people, we grieve and struggle while watching the disease destroy the person we once knew, torture, and kill them.

I cannot say losing a child is more challenging than losing somebody you've known for six to eight decades, an expression repeated a thousand times every time Juvenile Huntington's takes an infant or teenager. In some ways, it is more difficult to lose somebody you have known, loved, and depended on for decades, your entire life. Losing a loved one, young or old, hurts like hell.

But, when fatal diseases attack children, there is a more significant unfairness and leaves behind a lasting sting, creating a void too great to fill. We must prevent or cure this disease!

How Many People have Huntington's Disease?

Please understand that any numbers we provide are low because medical authorities often misdiagnose Huntington's disease for Parkinson's or Alzheimer's.

How Many Americans have Huntington's disease?

Each year, doctors diagnose 30,000 Americans with Huntington's disease, while over 200,000 are high risk[447].

How do the American numbers compare worldwide?

Let's review data by Stanford University to compare how many per million are getting Huntington's disease worldwide per million.

Black South Africa (.06), Japan (1-4), Hong Kong (3.7), and Finland (6.0) had the lowest incidents per million people.

Let's compare this to Europe (40-100), Northern Ireland (64), South Wales (76.1), Scotland (99.4), and the United States (100) incidents per million people[448].

These dramatic differences require more studies to figure out why European populations are much more likely to get Parkinson's disease than Asians or black Africans.

Is it the Western diet, lack of exercise, overuse of chemicals, and other environmental factors? The lack of sun exposure (and Vitamin D deficiencies) from European ancestors who drifted north? Is it because they misdiagnose Huntington's disease more in the third world?

The probable answer is all three, but it requires more studies to confirm. The disproportionate percentage of pale people living in western civilization getting Huntington's suggests a mysterious cause related to divergent evolution from eastern and darker cousins.

While I understand eastern civilization's reluctance to fund Huntington's disease research, I can only scratch my head, trying to rationalize why the western world does not invest greater into independent medical research to find a cure and means to prevent Huntington's disease.

What does Huntington's disease cost?

We divide costs into two categories, national and individual.

Annual Individual Huntington's disease costs

STAGE	ANNUAL COMMERCIAL COSTS	ANNUAL MEDICAID COSTS
Stage 1	$4,947	$3,257
Stage 2	$6,040	$5,670
Stage 3	$22,582	$27,111

Source: PubMed Study[449]

Please note the numbers are in 2013 dollars and are higher today.
When authorities provide newer data, I will update the numbers in the table.
Once again, we call on hospitals and medical authorities to form a digital link providing continuously updated medical information. We should have instant and accurate data, not aged and estimated numbers.

Huntington's Disease Symptoms

Huntington's disease, like other dementias, is a bully disease. Over the years, the torturous bully strips a person's ability to think, focus, reason, remember, balance, sit, or stand still, and everything that makes them a unique, vibrant individual.

"The hallmark symptom of Huntington's disease," explained Alzheimer's Association, "is uncontrolled movement of the arms, legs, head, face and upper body."

Let's put together a Huntington's symptoms list.

Huntington's disease symptoms list

- anger[450]
- anxiety[451]
- balance and posture trouble[452]
- concentration decline[453]
- convulsions of the head, face, arms, legs, and upper body[454]
- depression[455]
- deteriorating reasoning skills[456]
- impaired thinking[457]
- involuntary jerking[458]
- inability to plan and organize[459]

- irritable[460]
- memory problems[461]
- mood swings[462]
- personality changes
- speaking disturbances[463]
- swallowing disorder[464]
- unsteady gait
- weight loss[465]

Perhaps you noticed the similarities between this list and several other dementias, including Alzheimer's and Parkinson's disease. The similarities create confusion and often cause misdiagnosis.

A doctor must weigh the totality of symptoms, medical history, family history and order the tests to diagnose Huntington's disease.

Huntington's disease (HD)-related suicide

Let's discuss the elephant in the room. A disturbing topic but too important to ignore, suicide rates jump far higher in Huntington's disease patients than in general.

Most of Huntington's patients live their entire lives fearing HD, hoping the symptoms never appear, the diagnosis never comes.

The day arrives. In the period leading up to the diagnosis and at different intervals in the progression, it is vital to address depression and emotional issues.

According to the Huntington's Disease Society of America, the suicide rate for people with Huntington's disease is ten times the general population. A more recent study released in *Neurology* found Huntington's patients are twelve times more likely to commit suicide than those without HD.

HD suicide rate climbs up to twenty percent in pre-symptomatic patients and during certain stage intervals[466].

The Huntington's Disease Society of America recommends:

> *Monitor depression in the person with HD and ask about suicide regularly, as thoughts about death and suicide can be a part of depression. Suicide is of great concern in HD due to cognitive changes in the brain, including disinhibition and impulsivity*[467].

Patients, families, and medical professionals must understand the hopelessness, despair, and anxiety associated with Huntington's.

Emotional Support

Emotional support goes beyond the book's scope, but:

Open up to confidantes

When a neurological disorder strikes, we need to open up to our inner circle. HD is too complex a road to travel without people opening up and discussing what torments, emotionally or physically.

Mental health professionals

Once a neurologist diagnoses you or a loved one with Huntington's disease (HD), find a mental health professional to help navigate the emotional rollercoaster. Ask the neurologist or call the local Huntington's disease organizations and find one specializing in HD.

Remove weapons

Remove all weapons from the house, including any unnecessary medicine. Please do not make it easy to follow through on any suicidal thoughts associated with HD-induced depression and emotional problems.

If you love life, play it safe. The last thing we need when feeling suicidal is an easy and immediate path. Remove anything from the house making suicide potentially easy or fast.

Dances with Elephants

If doctors diagnose you with Huntington's disease, I recommend reading *Dancing with Elephants*[468] for emotional support and a roadmap to living with HD.

When diagnosed with Huntington's disease, Jarem Sawatsky refused to stop living. He turned to his family and developed a spiritual circle to develop a new reality of possibilities. Instead of allowing the idea of HD to defeat him before the severity of symptoms, he became an inspiration for the world.

One must not have HD to benefit from Sawatsky's beautifully written book. Still, Huntington's patients should read how Sawatsky thrived through kindness, laughter, and an inspiring determination to face each day, person, event, challenge, setback, and moment with a positive determination.

Dancing with Elephants galvanizes the soul and instills hope and courage. It is not a book about defeat, but the love of life and a strong will to make the best of whatever our challenges might be.

These ideas are but few to help fight HD-related emotional issues. Ask your mental health specialist for more ideas. Develop a plan to protect your life during darker moments.

Chapter 27: HYDROCEPHALUS

Let's begin our discussion by defining the word hydrocephalus. *Hydro*[169] means water, and *cephalus*[170] imply head.

The American Association of Neurological Surgeons describes hydrocephalus:

> *Hydrocephalus is a condition in which excess cerebrospinal fluid (CSF) builds up within the ventricles (fluid-containing cavities) of the brain and may increase pressure within the head. Although hydrocephalus described as "water on the brain," "the "water" is actually CSF, a clear fluid surrounding the brain and spinal cord. CSF has three crucial functions: 1) it acts as a "shock absorber" for the brain and spinal cord; 2) it acts as a vehicle for delivering nutrients to the brain and removing waste; and 3) it flows between the cranium and spine to regulate changes in pressure within the brain*[471].

Understanding hydrocephalus requires a basic knowledge of the brain, spinal cord, ventricles, and cerebrospinal fluid.

Let's view a hydrocephalus brain and see what causes the problem.

Hydrocephalus

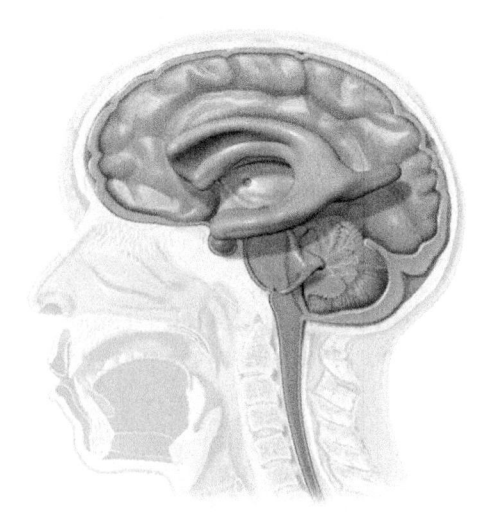

As you see in the image, too much cerebrospinal fluid bulges and damages the brain and spinal cord, causing hydrocephalus.

Primary hydrocephalus types

The two primary hydrocephalus types are communicating hydrocephalus and noncommunicating hydrocephalus. However, there are five other classifications:

- Normal pressure hydrocephalus
- Hydrocephalus ex-vacuo
- Acquired hydrocephalus
- Congenital hydrocephalus
- Compensated hydrocephalus

Communicating hydrocephalus

Our primary focus is communicating hydrocephalus (CH), or one of CH's subtypes, normal pressure hydrocephalus.

Medscape describes communicating hydrocephalus:

> *Communicating hydrocephalus occurs when full communication occurs between the ventricles and subarachnoid space. It is caused by overproduction of CSF (rarely), defective absorption of CSF (most often, includes conditions such as intracranial hemorrhage or meningitis resulting in damage to the arachnoid granulations, where CSF is reabsorbed), or venous drainage insufficiency (occasionally)*[472].

The primary communicating subtype is normal pressure hydrocephalus (NPHP), a proper name despite everybody's first reaction: *What's normal about hydrocephalus?*

Communicating normal pressure hydrocephalus

Medical authorities refer to hydrocephalus as communicating when cerebrospinal fluid flows uninterrupted through the brain's subarachnoid space and the ventricular system. Although rarer than Alzheimer's, Lewy body dementia, vascular dementia, and frontotemporal dementia, normal pressure hydrocephalus is another death-dealing disease. National Institute of Neurological Disorders and Stroke describes normal pressure hydrocephalus as one of the most mysterious dementias[473]:

> *Normal pressure hydrocephalus (NPH) is an abnormal buildup of cerebrospinal fluid (CSF) in the brain's ventricles, or cavities. It occurs if {something blocks} the normal flow of CSF throughout the brain and spinal cord. This causes the ventricles to enlarge, putting pressure on the brain. Normal*

pressure hydrocephalus can occur in people of any age, but it is most common in the elderly. It may result from a subarachnoid hemorrhage, head trauma, infection, tumor, or surgery complications. However, many people develop NPH even when none of these factors are present. In these cases, the cause of the disorder is unknown.

Since normal pressure hydrocephalus is a less prevalent form of dementia, it's likely to be years before we figure out these "unknown" causes.

Diagnosing normal pressure hydrocephalus is difficult because some symptoms overlap with Alzheimer's and other dementias. As every normal pressure hydrocephalus organization, researcher, or doctor attest, we need more funding for vital research.

We need to know the exact cause or causes to help develop urine or blood tests, vaccines, and cures.

Noncommunicating obstructive hydrocephalus

Unlike communicating between the ventricles and the subarachnoid space, noncommunicating or obstructive hydrocephalus occurs in the ventricle-connecting passages. Also known as obstructive hydrocephalus, noncommunicating hydrocephalus often occurs between the third and fourth ventricles in the Sylvius's aqueduct narrowing[474].

Doctors refer to hydrocephalus as non-communicating when a tumor or something blocks or inhibits cerebrospinal fluid in the ventricular system.

Other hydrocephalus classifications

There are four other hydrocephalus forms worth noting.

Hydrocephalus Ex-vacuo

This type results from traumatic brain injuries, stroke, or dementia such as Alzheimer's. Hydrocephalus ex-vacuo often shrinks brain tissue.

Acquired Hydrocephalus

Acquired normal pressure hydrocephalus occurs at or after birth.

Congenital Hydrocephalus

Babies with congenital normal pressure hydrocephalus are born with the disease.

Compensated hydrocephalus

Compensated hydrocephalus is present at birth or in early childhood but lingers, showing no symptoms into adulthood.

How many people have normal pressure hydrocephalus?

According to the Hydrocephalus Association, over 700,000 Americans suffer normal pressure hydrocephalus, but doctors often misdiagnose the symptoms as Parkinson's disease or Alzheimer's disease[475].

The number might be much higher.

According to the Cleveland Clinic[476], "as many as ten percent of people with dementia attributed to other disorders may actually have NPH {normal pressure hydrocephalus}."

Misdiagnosis

I blame misdiagnoses on four factors.

One, over 100 diseases are leading to dementia, and most share some symptoms. Two, with no blood or urine test for most, one cannot confirm the diagnosis for many dementias until postmortem during an autopsy. Three, there is not enough money to fund all the needed Alzheimer's studies, much less the lesser-known dementias, meaning we've barely broken the research surface for some. Four, diagnosing dementia is expensive and requires running imaging and other tests often not covered by insurance. Five, under training, incompetence causes some misdiagnosis, which is probably most serious under training.

Who gets normal pressure hydrocephalus?

Normal pressure hydrocephalus strikes most people over sixty[477] but attacks people of all ages, including newborns.

How many babies are born with normal pressure hydrocephalus?

Two of 1,000 babies are born with normal pressure hydrocephalus[478].

Is there a cure for normal pressure hydrocephalus?

Most dementias are incurable, but—if diagnosed early enough—the medical profession might reverse normal pressure hydrocephalus[479].

What are the medical costs for normal pressure hydrocephalus?

Normal pressure hydrocephalus medical costs surpass $2 billion per year[480].

What causes normal pressure hydrocephalus?

Researchers uncovered two pathways to normal pressure hydrocephalus:

1. Primary (idiopathic)
2. Secondary

Primary normal pressure hydrocephalus

If I hate the name normal pressure hydrocephalus, which I do, I profoundly dislike when we do not know the exact causes of neurological disorders. Normal Pressure Hydrocephalus cause remains unknown.

Secondary normal pressure hydrocephalus

Tumors, subarachnoid hemorrhages, and head injuries are the primary causes of this version[481].

Normal Pressure Hydrocephalus Symptoms (NPH)

Normal pressure hydrocephalus lacks the stages established for Alzheimer's and most dementias because it lags in research. Also, unlike other dementias, normal pressure hydrocephalus is often reversible. Therefore, it does not follow typical dementia stages.

We know the symptoms and, if untreated, grow more severe. Untreated or maltreated, normal pressure hydrocephalus causes premature death like most dementias.

As somebody who studies all the primary dementias, I enjoy researching normal pressure hydrocephalus. Not only do I find medical research fascinating, but there are positive outcomes.

If diagnosed and treated early, neurologists often reverse normal pressure hydrocephalus. Like anybody else, I love happy endings, and, overall, there are not enough of them in the dementia field.

Let's discuss the most common normal pressure hydrocephalus symptoms.

What are the symptoms of normal pressure hydrocephalus (NPH)?

Let's break down symptoms for primary and secondary NPH. This form leads to gait problems, urinary incontinence, and dementia[482].

The symptoms and progression differ from patient to patient, but below are typical.

- Attention-deficit[483]
- Bradyphrenia[484] (rigidity, weakness, tremors)
- Freezing (feeling as if one's feet stick to the floor)
- Impaired thinking skills[485]
- Inability to control the bladder (incontinence)[486]
- Irritability[487]
- Memory loss[488]
- Shuffled gait
- Walking difficulty[489]
- Injury from fall[490]

The gait and balance bladder issues are more pronounced in the beginning than cognitive issues[491].

Normal pressure hydrocephalus requires more studies, but this is one form of dementia that neurosurgeons can reduce through surgery if caught soon enough[492].

Unless examined by a neurosurgeon, doctors often misdiagnose normal pressure hydrocephalus.

Children and adults experience different normal pressure hydrocephalus. Because their fibrous joints connecting bones in the skull are not closed, children can better adapt to cerebrospinal fluid buildup than adults.

Most obvious normal pressure hydrocephalus symptoms for children

While children better adapt to the cerebrospinal fluid buildup, their heads grow unusually large.

Other normal pressure hydrocephalus symptoms for children

- Head soft spot bulges
- Skullbone gaps (split sutures)
- Irritability
- Seizures
- Sleepy
- Sun setting (Downward eyes)
- Swollen veins
- Vomiting

Normal pressure hydrocephalus symptoms for older children & adults

As we age, our heads and brains set, so the initial symptoms are more severe for older children and adults. Cerebrospinal fluid buildup puts pressure on the brain.

Older children and adults with normal pressure hydrocephalus first suffer headaches.

Other Normal Pressure Hydrocephalus Symptoms for Older Children & Adults

While they vary between patients, symptoms for adults and older children include physical, cognitive, and urinary issues.

- Blurred vision
- Depression
- Double vision
- Cognitive decline
- Drowsy
- Gait decline
- Impaired coordination
- Irritable
- Lethargic
- Memory loss
- Nausea
- Poor balance
- Sun setting
- Urinary incontinence
- Vomiting

Parkinson's disease and Creutzfeldt-Jakob share many symptoms, explaining why doctors often misdiagnose normal pressure hydrocephalus.

Symptoms Sources: American Association of Neurological Surgeons[493], Joseph H. Piatt Jr., MD[494], Child Neurology Foundation[495], Harvard Medical School[496], National Organization of Rare Disorders[497] (NORD), Johns Hopkins Medicine[498], National Health Service[499] (NHS).

Chapter 28: WERNICKE-KORSAKOFF SYNDROME

Some medical conditions happen to those with the healthiest habits, but bad habits are often responsible for Wernicke-Korsakoff.

Alcohol and tobacco have played star roles throughout our investigation of the dementias, and alcoholism is the force driving Wernicke-Korsakoff syndrome.

Alcoholism and other risk factors cause B1 deficiencies, damaging the brain's thalamus and hypothalamus, resulting in a severe memory disorder[500].

Wernicke-Korsakoff syndrome

According to American Addiction Center[501] (AAC):

> Wernicke-Korsakoff syndrome is a combination of two conditions in the brain caused by thiamine, or vitamin B1, deficiency: Wernicke's encephalopathy and Korsakoff syndrome or Korsakoff's psychosis. While they are separate conditions with different symptoms, they often co-occur, especially in people who have struggled with long-term alcohol dependence and abuse.

Let's examine Wernicke's encephalopathy and Korsakoff syndrome.

Wernicke's encephalopathy

In the first stage of Wernicke-Korsakoff Syndrome, Wernicke's encephalopathy causes acute symptoms that are life-threatening but often reversible if diagnosed early enough.

What is Wernicke's encephalopathy?

Sarayu Vasan, UCLA Kern Medical, and lead author of a Wernicke's Encephalopathy review released in *PubMed* described the disorder as follows[502]:

> Wernicke encephalopathy (WE) is an acute neurological condition characterized by a clinical triad of ophthalmoparesis with nystagmus, ataxia, and confusion. This is a life-threatening illness caused by thiamine deficiency, which primarily affects the peripheral and central nervous systems. {We should differentiate this} from Korsakoff syndrome, which is preventable and {often} a consequence of at least one episode of Wernicke's encephalopathy.

Korsakoff Syndrome

Damaging nerve cells supporting the spinal cord and brain, Korsakoff's syndrome is the chronic second stage where cognitive decline and other symptoms become far less reversible and often deadly.

The medical community debates whether Wernicke's encephalopathy always precedes Korsakoff syndrome. About 90% of Wernicke's encephalopathy patients develop Korsakoff syndrome[503], which explains the dementia category: Wernicke-Korsakoff syndrome.

What is Korsakoff syndrome?

Johns Hopkins Medicine describes Korsakoff syndrome as follows[504]:

> *Korsakoff's syndrome is a disorder that primarily affects the memory system in the brain. It usually results from a deficiency of thiamine (vitamin B1), {caused} by alcohol abuse, dietary deficiencies, prolonged vomiting, eating disorders, or the effects of chemotherapy.*

Since vitamin B deficiency causes both Wernicke and Korsakoff syndrome, let's analyze the connection.

Thiamine (vitamin B1)

Thiamine deficiency is front and center in every Wernicke and/or Korsakoff discussion.

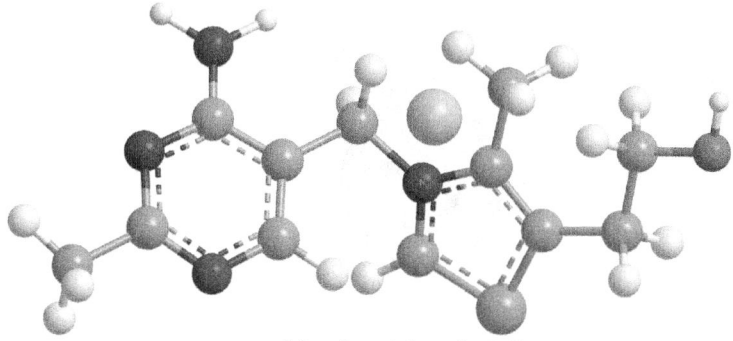

Thiamine (vitamin B1)

The Alzheimer's Association explains the connection[505].

> *Thiamine helps brain cells produce energy from sugar. When levels fall too low, brain cells cannot generate enough energy to function properly. Korsakoff syndrome is most commonly caused by alcohol misuse, but {also is} associated*

with AIDS, cancers that have spread throughout the body, chronic infections, poor nutrition and certain other conditions. It is also common in people whose bodies do not absorb food properly (malabsorption). This can sometimes occur with a chronic illness or after weight-loss (bariatric) surgery.

According to the NIH Office of Dietary Supplements, thiamin performs a crucial function in energy metabolism and developing and maintaining cells[506].

How many people have Wernicke-Korsakoff syndrome?

Wernicke-Korsakoff syndrome strikes 1-2.8 percent of Americans and is responsible for 59% of alcohol deaths[507].

Global prevalence

Wernicke-Korsakoff syndrome inflicts up to 4% of the French, about 3% of Australians, and up to 2% of the world population[508].

Who gets Wernicke-Korsakoff syndrome?

Wernicke-Korsakoff syndrome affects males somewhat more than females, and the disorder inflicts people between ages thirty and seventy in about equal proportions[509].

The disorder strikes senior citizens living alone, psychiatric patients, and the homeless in disproportionate numbers[510].

Is there a cure for Wernicke-Korsakoff syndrome?

Wernicke symptoms develop first and, if caught early enough, is reversible, but the chances decrease if it progresses to Wernicke-Korsakoff syndrome[511].

What causes Wernicke-Korsakoff syndrome?

Wernicke's encephalopathy and Korsakoff syndrome are independent disorders, but thiamine (vitamin B1) deficiency causes both.

Although not the only cause, alcohol is the primary cause of thiamine deficiency linked to Wernicke-Korsakoff Syndrome[512].

Other Causes

- AIDS
- Bariatric surgery
- Chemotherapy
- Colon cancer
- Deficient diet
- Eating disorders
- Gastric cancer

- Intestinal problems
- Kidney disorders
- Severe vomiting
- Stomach disorders

Sources: Alzheimer's Society of Canada[513], Penn State Neurology Center[514], Science Direct[515], University of Florida Health[516], Mount Sinai[517], *Journal of American Association*[518] (JAMA)

Ethanol/Alcohol

Ignoring alcohol abuse when discussing Wernick-Korsakoff syndrome is like ignoring the United States when talking about modern superpowers.

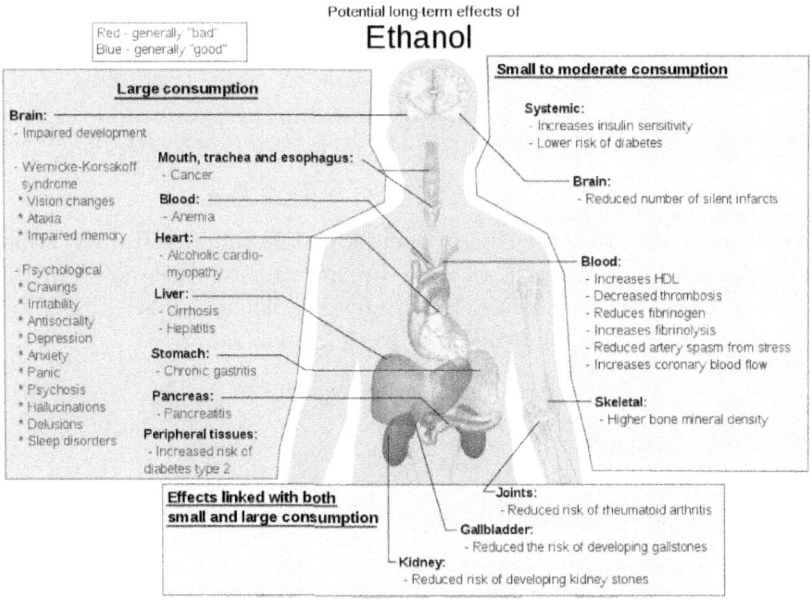

File: Possible long-term effects of ethanol.svg[519]

Alcohol is front and center in most Wernicke-Korsakoff syndrome cases. We understand why alcohol abuse ranks with tobacco as twin killers when we review the chart.

The image shows the damage alcohol inflicts, including impaired brain development, cancer to the mouth, esophagus, and trachea, anemia, cardiomyopathy, liver cirrhosis, hepatitis, chronic gastritis, pancreatitis, diabetes type 2, higher bone mineral deterioration, blood issues, several psychological issues, and several other health risks.

In the brain, alcohol causes a reduced number of silent infarcts. Alcohol also increases insulin sensitivity. Concerning Wernicke-Korsakoff syndrome, alcohol causes vision changes, ataxia, and impaired memory.

There are as many reasons not to abuse alcohol as excuses to do so, and we should do what we can to help brothers and sisters who abuse alcohol. However, be careful not to shame somebody diagnosed with alcohol-related Wernick-Korsakoff syndrome.

They stand wobbling at the fork in the road, determining whether they turn their lives around or drink themselves to premature death. The last thing they need is a bunch of: *I told you so this,* and *I told you so that.*

Wernicke-Korsakoff Syndrome Symptoms

According to Medscape, Wernicke-Korsakoff Syndrome most often "presents with the clinical triad of confusion, ataxia, and nystagmus[520]:"

> It is best conceptualized as 2 distinct syndromes, with one being characterized by an acute/subacute confusional state and often reversible findings of Wernicke encephalopathy (a type of delirium) and the other by persistent and irreversible findings of Korsakoff dementia.

According to the Alzheimer's Association, people suffering from Wernicke-Korsakoff syndrome "confabulate or make up, information they can't remember. They are not 'lying,' but may believe the invented explanations. Scientists don't yet understand why Korsakoff syndrome may cause confabulation[521]."

Wernicke-Korsakoff Syndrome Symptoms

- confusion[522]
- coma[523]
- double vision[524]
- decreased muscle coordination (ataxia)[525]
- gait abnormalities[526]
- hypothermia[527]
- Korsakoff's amnesic syndrome
- leg tremors[528]
- low blood pressure[529]
- memory loss[530]

See your doctor if you experience any symptoms. If caught early enough, Wernicke-Korsakoff syndrome is a (somewhat) reversible dementia if the patient overcomes their alcohol addiction.

If unrelated to alcohol abuse, genes or diet are the usual culprits. Patients should get to the doctor, and treatment should begin before the disorder progresses from Wernicke to Korsakoff syndrome.

There are two Wernicke-Korsakoff syndrome stages, and people should avoid stage two. At least 90% of alcoholic-related Wernicke-Korsakoff syndrome patients go from stage one to two.

I cannot overemphasize whether genes, an unhealthy diet, or alcohol abuse causes Wernicke; the only positive outcome is treating Wernicke before it develops to Korsakoff.

VIII. UPDATES

As part of our 2023 update, let's view some of the most important 2022 studies included in the companion book, *Dementia Research & News 1JAN2022 thru 1JAN2023*:

https://www.amazon.com/Dementia-Research-Overview-1JAN2022-1JAN2023/dp/B0BW2KMGYC

Chapter 29: HAVE WE BEEN BARKING UP THE WRONG TREE WITH BETA-AMYLOID PLAQUES THEORY?

Does Protein Buildup Cause Dementia?

We know a person is in neurological trouble when the cleaning process breaks down and protein accumulates in disproportionate numbers. Conventional wisdom argues that the protein turned rogue and causes Alzheimer's and other dementias.

We mentioned in the aphasia section how some neurologists challenge the idea and argue the protein buildup is a defensive attempt to protect the blame from the true cause.

A growing fraction within the neurological community challenges the amyloid cascade hypothesis, which claims rogue soluble beta-amyloid protein accumulates and forms amyloid plaques. While few challenge the damage the plaques cause to neurons and synapses, many suggest the protein is a defensive mechanism for the ever-elusive actual cause. If correct, this might explain why so many Alzheimer's drug trials fail.

Did Conventional Wisdom And The Mavericks Misunderstand The Role Of Protein Regarding Alzheimer's And Dementia?

A 2022 study focused on a new theory concerning the role of protein in dementia.

Researchers {Sturchio, Dwivedi, et al., 25OCT2022} tested their hypothesis that a decrease in soluble beta-amyloid is the actual cause of Alzheimer's symptoms.

Lead author Alberto Espay[531], MD, MSc, professor of neurology, University of Cincinnati, director and endowed chair of the James J. and Joan A. Gardner Family Center for Parkinson's Disease and Movement Disorders at the UC Gardner Neuroscience Institute and a UC Health physician, spoke about their hypothesis.

"The paradox is that so many of us accrue plaques in our brains as we age, and yet so few of us with plaques [develop] dementia," said Espay. "Yet the plaques remain the center of our attention as it relates to biomarker development and therapeutic strategies."

Getting Beyond The Paradox

First author Andrea Sturchio, MD, adjunct research instructor at UC's

College of Medicine, addressed this point.

"One of the strongest supports to the hypothesis of amyloid toxicity was based on these mutations," said Sturchio. "We studied that population because it offers the most important data."

Study Findings

"What we found," said Dr. Espay, "was that individuals already accumulating plaques in their brains who [can] generate high levels of soluble amyloid-beta have a lower risk of evolving into dementia over a three-year span."

The Meaning

"I think this is probably the best proof that reducing the level of the soluble form of the protein can be toxic," said Sturchio, "When done, patients have gotten worse."

Something We Lose, Not Something We Gain

"It's only too logical," said Espay, "if you are detached from the biases that we've created for too long, that a neurodegenerative process is caused by something we lose, amyloid-beta, rather than something we gain, amyloid plaques."

Dr. Espay and team combined neuroimaging and clinical assessments with a follow-up in 3.3 years, using the Clinical Dementia Rating scale to measure cognitive function and executive skills. They also measured beta-amyloid-42, p-tau, and t-tau cerebrospinal fluid levels.

A Process Of Loss

"Degeneration is a process of loss, and what we lose turns out to be much more important," said Dr. Espay.

Study Conclusion

The team[532] concluded:

> *Higher soluble Aβ$_{42}$ levels are associated with reduced risk of CDR progression, normal cognition, normal hippocampal volume, and normal precuneus metabolism to a greater extent than lower brain amyloid, lower p-tau, and lower t-tau levels in amyloid PiB-PET-positive individuals with autosomal dominant AD-causing genetic mutations. Brain toxicity in AD may be predominantly mediated by a*

reduction of the soluble protein pool, its functional fraction, rather than its accrual into amyloids.

Future studies should include a larger pool of participants and people with and without genetic Alzheimer's risk.

Chapter 30: DEMENTIA TESTING

I have lamented the lack of accurate, inexpensive testing for each dementia since I began researching neurological disorders many moons ago. Diagnosing dementia once the symptoms begin provides little to no means of reversing the disorder.

Testing is vital to developing lifestyle changes and medications to reverse these disorders before symptoms start. If we can diagnose dementia ten or twenty years before symptoms and learn the underlying causes, we can do more than treat symptoms, and perhaps prevent dementia from developing.

Several 2022 studies provide hope that one day soon, physicians can routinely test patients and recommend lifestyle changes and prescribe clinical treatment to prevent dementia.

Measuring Abdominal Aortic Calcification To Predict Dementia

An Edith Cowan University (ECU)-lead prospective study {Porter, Sim, et al., 26JUN2022} included 958 ambulant community-dwelling older women. The researchers measured abdominal aortic calcification (AAC) from lateral spine images (LSI) taken from a bone density machine to establish a 1998 baseline. The team monitored the women's health for fifteen years.

The researchers categorized abdominal aortic calcification:
- Low
- Moderate
- Extensive

Half of the women developed medium to high abdominal aortic calcification (AFF) levels and were twice as likely to develop dementia as those with lower AAC levels.

"There's an adage in dementia research that what's good for your heart is good for your brain," said Simon Laws[533], professor and director of the Centre for Precision Health. "This study reaffirms this link and further adds to our understanding of late-onset dementia risk and potential preventative strategies."

How so?

"What's come to light is the importance of modifying risk factors such as diet and physical activity in preventing dementia," said Laws. "You need to intervene early, and hopefully, this study allows for the earliest possible change and the greatest impact."

Laws said abdominal aortic calcification (ACC) helps identify fifty percent of people who will develop Alzheimer's.

Study Conclusion

The team[534] concluded:

> This study identified an association between AAC and the subsequent development of late-life dementia. Significant increases in risk for hospitalization and death from dementia were observed with increasing severity of AAC, [and] to shorter times to each of these events. Several proposed mechanisms and pathways [impacted] by an individual's cardiovascular risk profile likely contribute to the relationship between AAC and dementia. Therefore, understanding the impact of shared risk factors could allow for targeted disease-modifying strategies. To this end, lateral spine imaging to detect AAC [and] spine fractures during bone density

scanning has [the] potential for use as an early screening and assessment tool to identify women at higher risk of dementia, allowing for [implementing] early lifestyle intervention strategies in at-risk populations. Such studies should be a high priority for long-term randomised controlled trials.

Low Muscle Mass And Cognitive Decline

A cohort study {Tessier, Wing, et al., 1JUL2023} investigated the association between low muscle mass and cognitive decline. The researchers analyzed data from 8,279 older people over three years.

Lead author Stéphanie Chevalier[535], a Metabolic Disorders and Complications Program scientist at the Research Institute of the McGill University Health Centre, addressed their results.

"Low muscle strength has been recently associated with [a] greater risk of dementia," said Chevalier, "but little is known about a possible link between muscle mass and cognition."

Dr. Chevalier and team analyzed data from the Canadian Longitudinal Study on Aging (CLSA), which measures body composition and cognitive health every three years.

"With this study," said Chevalier, "we show for the first time [that] low muscle mass is significantly associated with faster cognitive decline and that this association is independent of muscle strength and physical activity level, among other factors."

What makes your findings important?

"Because muscle mass is a modifiable factor, [we] can do something about it," said Chevalier. "Exercise—particularly resistance exercise—and good nutrition with sufficient protein can help maintain muscle mass over the years."

Study Conclusion

The team[536] concluded:

> This cohort study found [that] low muscle mass measured by DXA was significantly and independently associated with faster subsequent executive function decline over three years among adults aged at least 65 years. Importantly, DXA is widely available, and measures of lean mass could be routinely incorporated into the image analyses. Clinical screening of older adults to identify those with low muscle mass may provide insight regarding their risk of developing cognitive impairment [and] guide the testing and application of preventative or therapeutic interventions.

The study raises the possibility of testing older people for muscle mass loss to determine the risk of cognitive decline and dementia. Considering other studies showed a link between reduced muscle strength and dementia risk, this study's results are consistent. Muscle health and mental well-being appear linked.

CONCLUSION

Thank you for reading this book. We covered a good amount of material.

Dementia is a cruel neurological disorder that robs people of their personalities, executive skills, memories, talents, language, voice, motor capabilities, and all that makes us individuals.

Alzheimer's and Dementia

Although Alzheimer's disease (AD) is the most prevalent, we learned AD is to dementia what China is to Asia. Alzheimer's represents 60-80% of dementia, but 19 dementia types account for 99 percent.

Dementia Spares No Demographic

Known as an old folk disease, dementia strikes people of all ages. Most dementia is not genetic, although certain types such as Huntington's disease are 100% familial.

Dementia is irreversible.

Unlike most dementia, neurological surgeons can treat and sometimes reverse normal pressure hydrocephalus if caught early enough.

Dementia Prevalence

The first section focused on dementia as a general category. We learned 850,000 people in the UK have dementia, compared to 5.8 Americans and 50 million people worldwide.

Dementia Categories

We divided the 19 dementias into six categories:

- Lewy Body/Parkinsonism related dementias
- Alzheimer's related dementias
- Frontotemporal lobar degeneration related dementias
- Primary progressive aphasia related dementias
- Vascular dementias
- Other dementias

Of the 19 dementias, several are subtypes, but this work extends each equal status and inquiry.

Lewy Body/Parkinsonism Related Dementias
1. Dementia with Lewy bodies
2. Parkinson's disease dementia

Frontotemporal Lobar Degeneration Related Dementias
3. Behavioral variant frontotemporal dementia
4. Progressive supranuclear palsy

Primary Progressive Aphasia Related Dementias
5. Nonfluent primary progressive aphasia (nPPA)
6. Logopenic progressive aphasia (lPPA)
7. Semantic primary progressive aphasia (sPPA)

Vascular Dementia
8. Cortical vascular dementia
9. Binswanger disease

Alzheimer's Related Dementias
10. Alzheimer's disease (Including Down syndrome with AD)
11. Posterior cortical atrophy
12. Limbic-predominant age-related TDP-43 encephalopathy (LATE)

Other Dementias
13. Normal pressure hydrocephalus
14. Huntington's disease
15. Korsakoff syndrome
16. Creutzfeldt-Jakob disease
17. Amyotrophic lateral sclerosis
18. Corticobasal syndrome
19. Chronic traumatic encephalopathy

We examined each dementia type, defining and exploring history, causes, prevalence, and symptoms.

Can Computer Processing Software Detect Cognitive Decline?

I've agonized in every dementia book I've written over the lack of blood and urine tests to detect dementia, especially before symptoms begin. While researchers continue working to develop blood or urine testing, none appear close to complete development, much less FDA (or equivalent) approval.

Researchers do not limit the effort to blood and urine tests, as several innovative scientists look to our senses and ways to measure the sense of smell, hearing, and vision. How about voice?

Boston University researchers {Hao, Song, et al., 7JUL2022} created a voice analyzation tool to diagnose cognitive decline and Alzheimer's disease.

Co-author Ioannis Paschalidis[537], a BU College of Engineering Distinguished Professor of Engineering and director of BU's Rafik B. Hariri Institute for Computing and Computational Science & Engineering, said, "This approach brings us one step closer to early intervention."

Dr. Paschalidis emphasized that quicker Alzheimer's diagnosis would inspire dozens of studies on intervention techniques and drugs to reverse or slow cognitive degeneration.

"It can form the basis of an online tool that could reach everyone," said Paschalidis, "and could increase the number of people who get screened early."

Audio features did not provide a significant distinction to help identify cognitive impairment and dementia. Transcribed interviews proved far more critical.

"It surprised us that speech flow or other audio features are not that critical," said Paschalidis. "You can automatically transcribe interviews reasonably well and rely on text analysis through AI to assess cognitive impairment."

Study Conclusion

The team[538] concluded:

> *The proposed approach offers a fully automated identification of MCI and dementia based on a recorded neuropsychological test, providing an opportunity to develop a remote screening tool that could be adapted easily to any language.*

"Our models can help clinicians assess patients in terms of their chances of cognitive decline," said Paschalidis, "and then best tailor resources to them by doing further testing on those [with] a higher likelihood of dementia."

Developing simple, quick, inexpensive, and accurate tests for Alzheimer's and other dementias remains a priority in the dream of significantly minimizing, if not defeating, dementia. It will be interesting to see where the work of Dr. Paschalidis and his team leads.

Can Urine Biomarker Detect Early Dementia?

Having pined for a simple urine test to detect dementia years before the symptoms began, a Chinese study caught my eye.

Shanghai Jiao Tong University {Wang, Wang, et al., 30NOV2022} investigated urinary formic acid's association with Alzheimer's plasma biomarkers.

The team divided 574 participants into five groups:
- Normal cognition/71 participants
- Subjective cognitive decline/101 participants
- Cognitive impairment minus mild cognitive impairment/131 participants
- Mild cognitive impairment/158 participants
- Diagnosed with Alzheimer's disease/113 participants

The Results

Compared to healthy controls, the team discovered increased urinary formic acid levels in all Alzheimer's groups.

The research team said, "Urinary formic acid and formaldehyde are [likely] new biomarkers independent of the existing AD diagnostic criteria."

The Implications

"Using these urine biomarkers can significantly promote the popularity of early screening for AD," said the research team, "which can improve advice on diagnosis, treatment, and lifestyle for people at risk for AD."

Study Conclusion

The team[539] concluded:

> In conclusion, urinary formic acid levels changed dynamically, related to the deterioration of cognitive function. Urinary formaldehyde levels were related to [the] APOE ε4 genotype and the presence of Aβ depositions in the brain. Urinary formic acid and formaldehyde levels could not only be used for differentiation between AD and NC but also could improve the prediction accuracy of plasma biomarkers for disease stages of AD. Our systematic evaluation revealed the novel possibility of urinary formic acid as a potential biomarker for the early diagnosis of AD.

The researchers called for further investigations to develop diagnostic models to gauge urinary formic acid and formaldehyde levels. The team argued urine testing provides "unique advantages in early screening in the community."

Can Drawing Process Indicate Which Type Of Dementia?

Japanese researchers from the University of Tsukuba[540] and IBM Research {Yasunori, Masatomo, et al., 8NOV2022} analyzed drawing tests using electronic tablets and pens for patients to compare participants with dementia with Lewy bodies (DLB) and Alzheimer's disease (AD).

The team focused on distinguishing between three neurological disorders:
- Alzheimer's disease
- Dementia with Lewy bodies
- Parkinson's disease

*When Parkinson's disease develops dementia, and dementia with Lewy bodies develops Parkinson's symptoms, they become the same in clinical terms. Dementia with Lewy bodies begins with dementia, and Parkinson's disease dementia is Parkinson's disease unless they develop dementia symptoms.

The Results

Professor Tetsuaki Arai, the Senior Author, reported their findings.

"Different drawing tasks played determinant roles in classifying different pairs of these three diagnostic groups," said Ari. "This is the first study to highlight the usefulness of combining multiple drawing tasks for enabling both identification and differentiation of AD and DLB."

Study Conclusion

The team[541] concluded:

> Our results provide initial evidence of (i) discriminative differences in features characterizing the drawing process that would reflect cognitive and motor impairments in AD and DLB and (ii) the feasibility of machine-learning models using these features to identify and differentiate AD and DLB. Specifically, we identified particular features and drawing tasks that could facilitate either the identification or differentiation of AD and DLB and [the] effective combination of those features and tasks could enable identification and differentiation. A future study is needed [to understand better] the applicability of our findings to clinical practice [and] other forms of Lewy body disorders and related diseases.

The team next wants to discover drawing impairment signatures to identify and distinguish Alzheimer's and dementia with Lewy bodies.

Predicting Dementia Nine Years Before First Symptoms

Researchers {Swaddiwudhipong, Whiteside, et al., 12OCT2022} investigated UK Biobank data in search of cognitive and functional measures before diagnosis for:
- Alzheimer's disease (AD)
- Frontotemporal dementia (FTD)
- Dementia with Lewy bodies (DLB)
- Multiple system atrophy
- Parkinson's disease (PD)
- Progressive supranuclear palsy (PSP)

The team compared the measures for the above neurological disorders to participants without neurodegeneration.

The Goal

Senior author Dr. Tim Rittman from the Department of Clinical Neurosciences at the University of Cambridge[542] said:

The problem with clinical trials is that, by necessity, they often recruit patients with a diagnosis, but we know that by this point, they are already some way down the road, and their condition cannot be stopped. If we can find these individuals early enough, we'll have a better chance of seeing if the drugs are effective.

The team analyzed information from 500,000 participants in the UK Biobank aged forty to sixty-nine to determine symptoms before dementia diagnosis.

The Results

First author Nol Swaddiwudhipong, a junior doctor at the University of Cambridge, spoke about the study.

"When we looked back at patients' histories, it became clear that they were showing some cognitive impairment several years before their symptoms became obvious enough to prompt a diagnosis," said Swaddiwudhipong. "The impairments were often subtle, but across [several] aspects of cognition."

The Importance

"This is a step towards us being able to screen people [at] greatest risk," said Swaddiwudhipong. "For example, people over 50 or those who have high blood pressure or do not do enough exercise—and intervene at an earlier stage to help them reduce their risk."

Study Conclusion

The team[543] concluded:

The scale and longitudinal follow-up of UK Biobank

participants provide evidence for cognitive and functional decline years before symptoms become obvious in multiple neurodegenerative diseases. Identifying pre-diagnostic functional and cognitive changes could improve selection for preventive and early disease-modifying treatment trials.

The study shows it is possible to identify dementia up to nine years before diagnosis.

THE END

Of

2022 DEMENTIA OVERVIEW

ABOUT THE AUTHOR.

Jerry Beller is the lead author and researcher at Beller Medical Research. Beller distinguished himself by breaking medical ground three times.

He wrote the first book covering all 15 primary dementia types, which he since expanded to cover nineteen. Beller followed this accomplishment by writing a book on each dementia type. He broke medical ground a third time when he published the first book on the new dementia category, LATE.

When the world struggled to grasp the difference between Alzheimer's disease and China, Beller explained:

> *Alzheimer's is only one dementia, much like China is only one country in Asia. Just as we do not want to ignore the other countries in Asia because China is the largest, nor do we want to ignore the less prevalent dementia types.*

Despite his accomplishments, he remains humble. "Until we win the dementia war, I've no reason to celebrate," Beller said. "If we win the war during my lifetime, I will celebrate with a few hundred brothers and sisters around the world who share my passion. Until then, we have too much work left to worry about accolades and legacies."

When not researching dementia, Jerry enjoys life with his wife of thirty-plus years, Nicola, and their two children.

Visit Jerry Beller:
https://bellerhealth.com

[1] 'Dementia More Feared than Cancer New Saga Survey Reveals', *Saga* <https://newsroom.saga.co.uk/news/dementia-more-feared-than-cancer-new-saga-survey-reveals> [accessed 22 November 2021].

[2] 'Alzheimer's Disease Facts and Figures', *Alzheimer's Disease and Dementia* <https://www.alz.org/alzheimers-dementia/facts-figures> [accessed 21 March 2022].

[3] 'Alzheimer's Disease Facts and Figures'.

[4] Ronald C. Petersen and others, 'Practice Guideline Update Summary: Mild Cognitive Impairment: Report of the Guideline Development, Dissemination, and Implementation Subcommittee of the American Academy of Neurology', *Neurology*, 90.3 (2018), 126–35 <https://doi.org/10.1212/WNL.0000000000004826>.

[5] 'Lewy Body Dementia - Symptoms and Causes - Mayo Clinic' <https://www.mayoclinic.org/diseases-conditions/lewy-body-dementia/symptoms-causes/syc-20352025> [accessed 18 February 2018].

[6] 'What Is LBD? | Lewy Body Dementia Association' <https://www.lbda.org/category/3437/what-is-lbd.htm> [accessed 18 February 2018].

[7] 'Parkinson's Disease Dementia', *Memory and Aging Center* <https://memory.ucsf.edu/parkinson-disease-dementia> [accessed 24 April 2019].

[8] Suraj Rajan, *English: Photomicrograph of Regions of Substantia Nigra in a Parkinson's Patient Showing Lewy Bodies and Lewy Neurites in Various Magnifications. Top Panels Show a 60-Times Magnification of the Alpha Synuclein Intraneuronal Inclusions Aggregated to Form Lewy Bodies. The Bottom Panels Are 20 × Magnification Images That Show Strand-like Lewy Neurites and Rounded Lewy Bodies of Various Sizes. Neuromelanin Laden Cells of the Substantia Nigra Are Visible in the Background. Stains Used: Mouse Monoclonal Alpha-Synuclein Antibody; Counterstained with Mayer's Haematoxylin.*, 2012, Own work <https://commons.wikimedia.org/wiki/File:Lewy_bodies_(alpha_synuclein_inclusions).svg> [accessed 23 April 2019].

[9] 'A New Insight into Parkinson's Disease Protein | UC San Francisco', *A New Insight into Parkinson's Disease Protein | UC San Francisco* <https://www.ucsf.edu/news/2017/07/407866/new-insight-parkinsons-disease-protein> [accessed 24 April 2019].

[10] 'Chapter 11: The Cerebral Cortex' <https://www.dartmouth.edu/~rswenson/NeuroSci/chapter_11.html> [accessed 24 April 2019].

[11] 'Human Brain', *Wikipedia*, 2019 <https://en.wikipedia.org/w/index.php?title=Human_brain&oldid=893696243> [accessed 24 April 2019].

[12] T. Huff and S. C. Dulebohn, 'Neuroanatomy, Visual Cortex', 2018 <http://europepmc.org/abstract/med/29494110> [accessed 24 April 2019].

[13] 'ASSOCIATION CORTEX' <http://www.indiana.edu/~p1013447/dictionary/assn_cor.htm> [accessed 24 April 2019].

[14] 'Know Your Brain: Primary Somatosensory Cortex — Neuroscientifically Challenged' <https://neuroscientificallychallenged.com/blog/know-your-brain-primary-somatosensory-cortex> [accessed 24 April 2019].

[15] Simon B. Eickhoff and others, 'Anatomical and Functional Connectivity of Cytoarchitectonic Areas within the Human Parietal Operculum', *The Journal of Neuroscience: The Official Journal of the Society for Neuroscience*, 30.18 (2010), 6409–21 <https://doi.org/10.1523/JNEUROSCI.5664-09.2010>.

[16] Fritzie I. Arce-McShane and others, 'Primary Motor and Sensory Cortical Areas Communicate via Spatiotemporally Coordinated Networks at Multiple Frequencies', *Proceedings of the National Academy of Sciences of the United States of America*, 113.18 (2016), 5083–88 <https://doi.org/10.1073/pnas.1600788113>.

[17] *Neuroscience*, 2nd edn (Sinauer Associates, 2001).

[18] Lutz Jäncke, Marcus Cheetham, and Thomas Baumgartner, 'Virtual Reality and the Role of the Prefrontal Cortex in Adults and Children.', *Frontiers in Neuroscience*, 3 (2009) <https://doi.org/10.3389/neuro.01.006.2009>.

[19] 'Lewy Body Dementias', *Memory and Aging Center* <https://memory.ucsf.edu/lewy-body-dementias> [accessed 24 April 2019].

[20] 'Dementia with Lewy Bodies (DLB) | Johns Hopkins Medicine' <https://www.hopkinsmedicine.org/health/conditions-and-diseases/dementia/dementia-with-lewy-bodies> [accessed 24 April 2019].

[21] 'What Is LBD? | Lewy Body Dementia Association' <https://www.lbda.org/go/what-lbd-0> [accessed 24 April 2019].

[22] '10 Things You Should Know about LBD | Lewy Body Dementia Association' <https://www.lbda.org/go/10-things-you-should-know-about-lbd> [accessed 24 April 2019].

[23] Yoshio Tsuboi and Dennis W. Dickson, 'Dementia with Lewy Bodies and Parkinson's Disease with Dementia: Are They Different?', *Parkinsonism & Related Disorders*, 11 Suppl 1 (2005), S47-51 <https://doi.org/10.1016/j.parkreldis.2004.10.014>.

[24] 'This Month in Physics History' <http://www.aps.org/publications/apsnews/200502/history.cfm> [accessed 3 December 2020].

[25] 'Einstein's Theory of Special Relativity | Space' <https://www.space.com/36273-theory-special-relativity.html> [accessed 3 December 2020].

[26] 'Einstein's Explanation Of Photoelectric Effect - Threshold Frequency | BYJU'S', *BYJUS* <https://byjus.com/physics/einsteins-explaination/> [accessed 3 December 2020].

[27] 'Mass-Energy Equivalence', *Physics LibreTexts*, 2016 <https://phys.libretexts.org/Bookshelves/Relativity/Supplemental_Modules_(Relativity)/Miscellaneous_Relativity_Topics/Mass-Energy_Equivalence> [accessed 3 December 2020].

[28] 'Suman Mulumudi | Columbia Engineering'

<https://www.engineering.columbia.edu/egleston-scholars/suman-mulumudi> [accessed 3 December 2020].

[29] 'What Did Galileo Invent? - Universe Today' <https://www.universetoday.com/48758/galileo-inventions/> [accessed 3 December 2020].

[30] Desmond Clarke, 'Blaise Pascal', in *The Stanford Encyclopedia of Philosophy*, ed. by Edward N. Zalta, Fall 2015 (Metaphysics Research Lab, Stanford University, 2015) <https://plato.stanford.edu/archives/fall2015/entries/pascal/> [accessed 3 December 2020].

[31] 'Friedrich Heinrich Lewy Body Dementia Lewey Frederic Shaking Palsy Paralysis Agitans Parkinson Hans Förstl' <http://www2.psykl.med.tum.de/geschichte_history/lewy1991.html> [accessed 6 January 2019].

[32] Bernd Holdorff, 'Friedrich Heinrich Lewy (1885-1950) and His Work', *Journal of the History of the Neurosciences*, 11.1 (2002), 19–28 <https://doi.org/10.1076/jhin.11.1.19.9106>.

[33] Ana Maria Cuervo and others, 'Impaired Degradation of Mutant Alpha-Synuclein by Chaperone-Mediated Autophagy', *Science (New York, N.Y.)*, 305.5688 (2004), 1292–95 <https://doi.org/10.1126/science.1101738>.

[34] Ajpolino, *English: A Structural Model of Human Alpha-Synuclein Using Data from Ulmer TS, Bax A, Cole NB, Nussbaum RL (2005). J Biol Chem 280:9595-9603. DOI: 10.1074/Jbc.M411805200 Accessed from the Protein Data Bank at Https://Www.Rcsb.Org/Structure/1XQ8 and Modeled Using PyMOL.*, 2020, Own work <https://commons.wikimedia.org/wiki/File:Alpha-synuclein_2005.png> [accessed 23 September 2020].

[35] K Uéda and others, 'Molecular Cloning of CDNA Encoding an Unrecognized Component of Amyloid in Alzheimer Disease.', *Proceedings of the National Academy of Sciences of the United States of America*, 90.23 (1993), 11282–86.

[36] Vladimir N. Uversky, 'A Protein-Chameleon: Conformational Plasticity of Alpha-Synuclein, a Disordered Protein Involved in Neurodegenerative Disorders', *Journal of Biomolecular Structure & Dynamics*, 21.2 (2003), 211–34 <https://doi.org/10.1080/07391102.2003.10506918>.

[37] Mark R. Cookson, *English: Events in α-Synuclein Toxicity. The Central Panel Shows the Major Pathway for Protein Aggregation. Monomeric α-Synuclein Is Natively Unfolded in Solution but Can Also Bind to Membranes in an α-Helical Form. It Seems Likely That These Two Species Exist in Equilibrium within the Cell, Although This Is Unproven. From in Vitro Work, It Is Clear That Unfolded Monomer Can Aggregate First into Small Oligomeric Species That Can Be Stabilized by β-Sheet-like Interactions and Then into Higher Molecular Weight Insoluble Fibrils. In a Cellular Context, There Is Some Evidence That the Presence of Lipids Can Promote Oligomer Formation: α-Synuclein Can Also Form Annular, Pore-like Structures That Interact with Membranes. The Deposition of α-Synuclein into Pathological Structures Such as Lewy Bodies Is Probably a Late Event That Occurs in Some Neurons. On the Left Hand Side Are Some of the Known Modifiers of This Process. Electrical Activity in Neurons Changes the Association of α-Synuclein with Vesicles and May Also Stimulate Polo-like Kinase 2 (PLK2), Which Has Been Shown*

to Phosphorylate α-Synuclein at Ser129. Other Kinases Have Also Been Proposed to Be Involved. As Well as Phosphorylation, Truncation through Proteases Such as Calpains, and Nitration, Probably through Nitric Oxide (NO) or Other Reactive Nitrogen Species That Are Present during Inflammation, All Modify Synuclein Such That It Has a Higher Tendency to Aggregate. The Addition of Ubiquitin (Shown as a Black Spot) to Lewy Bodies Is Probably a Secondary Process to Deposition. On the Right Are Some of the Proposed Cellular Targets for α-Synuclein Mediated Toxicity, Which Include (from Top to Bottom) ER-Golgi Transport, Synaptic Vesicles, Mitochondria and Lysosomes and Other Proteolytic Machinery. In Each of These Cases, It Is Proposed That α-Synuclein Has Detrimental Effects, Listed below Each Arrow, Although at This Time It Is Not Clear If Any of These Are Either Necessary or Sufficient for Toxicity in Neurons. Cookson Molecular Neurodegeneration 2009 4:9 Doi:10.1186/1750-1326-4-9, 2009, α-Synuclein and neuronal cell death <https://commons.wikimedia.org/wiki/File:Events_in_alpha_synuclein_toxicity.jpg> [accessed 22 September 2020].

[38] Mark R. Cookson, 'α-Synuclein and Neuronal Cell Death', *Molecular Neurodegeneration*, 4.1 (2009), 9 <https://doi.org/10.1186/1750-1326-4-9>.

[39] Thomas Splettstoesser, *English: Schematic of a Synapse*, 2015, Own work <https://commons.wikimedia.org/wiki/File:SynapseSchematic_en.svg> [accessed 22 September 2020].

[40] Doris L. Fortin and others, 'Lipid Rafts Mediate the Synaptic Localization of Alpha-Synuclein', *The Journal of Neuroscience: The Official Journal of the Society for Neuroscience*, 24.30 (2004), 6715–23 <https://doi.org/10.1523/JNEUROSCI.1594-04.2004>.

[41] A. Iwai and others, 'The Precursor Protein of Non-A Beta Component of Alzheimer's Disease Amyloid Is a Presynaptic Protein of the Central Nervous System', *Neuron*, 14.2 (1995), 467–75 <https://doi.org/10.1016/0896-6273(95)90302-x>.

[42] P. J. Kahle and others, 'Subcellular Localization of Wild-Type and Parkinson's Disease-Associated Mutant Alpha -Synuclein in Human and Transgenic Mouse Brain', *The Journal of Neuroscience: The Official Journal of the Society for Neuroscience*, 20.17 (2000), 6365–73.

[43] 'Scientists Identify New Target for Parkinson's Therapies' <https://medicalxpress.com/news/2020-03-scientists-parkinson-therapies.html> [accessed 25 September 2020].

[44] 'Dementia with Lewy Bodies (DLB)', *Cedars-Sinai* <https://www.cedars-sinai.org/health-library/diseases-and-conditions/d/dementia-with-lewy-bodies-dlb.html> [accessed 24 April 2019].

[45] 'Dementia with Lewy Bodies Symptoms| Signs, Symptoms, & Diagnosis', *Dementia* <//www.alz.org/dementia/dementia-with-lewy-bodies-symptoms.asp> [accessed 18 February 2018].

[46] Bernd Holdorff, 'Centenary of Tretiakoff's Thesis on the Morphology of Parkinson's Disease, Evolved on the Grounds of Encephalitis Lethargica Pathology', *Journal of the History of the Neurosciences*, 28.4 (2019), 387–98 <https://doi.org/10.1080/0964704X.2019.1622361>.

[47] 'SNCA Gene: MedlinePlus Genetics' <https://medlineplus.gov/genetics/gene/snca/> [accessed 3 December 2020].

[48] I. G. McKeith and others, 'Consensus Guidelines for the Clinical and Pathologic Diagnosis of Dementia with Lewy Bodies (DLB): Report of the Consortium on DLB International Workshop', *Neurology*, 47.5 (1996), 1113–24 <https://doi.org/10.1212/wnl.47.5.1113>.

[49] 'Dementia with Lewy Bodies Consortium', *Wikipedia*, 2020 <https://en.wikipedia.org/w/index.php?title=Dementia_with_Lewy_Bodies_Consortium&oldid=956652057> [accessed 2 December 2020].

[50] 'Lewy Body Dementia Is a Life-Shortening, Terminal Diagnosis', *BioSpace* <https://www.biospace.com/article/lewy-body-dementia-is-a-life-shortening-terminal-diagnosis/> [accessed 19 October 2020].

[51] 'What Is Dementia with Lewy Bodies?', *Alzheimer's Research UK* <https://www.alzheimersresearchuk.org/dementia-information/types-of-dementia/dementia-with-lewy-bodies/> [accessed 20 October 2020].

[52] Joseph P. M. Kane and others, 'Clinical Prevalence of Lewy Body Dementia', *Alzheimer's Research & Therapy*, 10 (2018) <https://doi.org/10.1186/s13195-018-0350-6>.

[53] Sheng-Kung Yang and others, 'Incidence and Comorbidity of Dementia with Lewy Bodies: A Population-Based Cohort Study', *Behavioural Neurology* (Hindawi, 2018), e7631951 <https://doi.org/10.1155/2018/7631951>.

[54] 'Alzheimers-Facts-and-Figures-2019-r.Pdf' <https://www.alz.org/media/documents/alzheimers-facts-and-figures-2019-r.pdf> [accessed 20 October 2020].

[55] Ian McKeith, 'Dementia with Lewy Bodies', *Dialogues in Clinical Neuroscience*, 6.3 (2004), 333–41.

[56] '49-12616-6416-723.Pdf' <https://www.aapm.org/meetings/amos2/pdf/49-12616-6416-723.pdf> [accessed 20 October 2020].

[57] 'Dementia with Lewy Bodies', *Department of Neurology*, 2020 <https://www.columbianeurology.org/neurology/staywell/dementia-lewy-bodies> [accessed 20 October 2020].

[58] Victor W Henderson, 'Dementia with Lewy Bodies', *Dementia with Lewy Bodies*, 6.

[59] 'Vascular Dementia | Johns Hopkins Medicine' <https://www.hopkinsmedicine.org/health/conditions-and-diseases/dementia/vascular-dementia> [accessed 20 October 2020].

[60] 'Vascular Dementia' <https://stanfordhealthcare.org/medical-conditions/brain-and-nerves/dementia/types/vascular-dementia.html> [accessed 20 October 2020].

[61] 'Vascular Dementia: What Is It, and What Causes It?', *Alzheimer's Society* <https://www.alzheimers.org.uk/about-dementia/types-dementia/vascular-dementia>

[accessed 20 October 2020].

[62] Gustavo C. Román, 'Vascular Dementia May Be the Most Common Form of Dementia in the Elderly', *Journal of the Neurological Sciences*, 203–204 (2002), 7–10 <https://doi.org/10.1016/s0022-510x(02)00252-6>.

[63] '10 Things You Need to Know about Lewy Body Dementia | Lewy Body Dementia Association' <https://www.lbda.org/content/10-things-you-need-know-about-lewy-body-dementia> [accessed 18 February 2018].

[64] Ursula Hohl and others, 'Diagnostic Accuracy of Dementia With Lewy Bodies', *Archives of Neurology*, 57.3 (2000), 347 <https://doi.org/10.1001/archneur.57.3.347>.

[65] Alan J. Thomas and others, 'Improving the Identification of Dementia with Lewy Bodies in the Context of an Alzheimer's-Type Dementia', *Alzheimer's Research & Therapy*, 10 (2018) <https://doi.org/10.1186/s13195-018-0356-0>.

[66] Tomoya Kon, Masahiko Tomiyama, and Koichi Wakabayashi, 'Neuropathology of Lewy Body Disease: Clinicopathological Crosstalk between Typical and Atypical Cases', *Neuropathology*, 40.1 (2020), 30–39 <https://doi.org/10.1111/neup.12597>.

[67] Caroline Bouter and others, 'Case Report: The Role of Neuropsychological Assessment and Imaging Biomarkers in the Early Diagnosis of Lewy Body Dementia in a Patient With Major Depression and Prolonged Alcohol and Benzodiazepine Dependence', *Frontiers in Psychiatry*, 11 (2020) <https://doi.org/10.3389/fpsyt.2020.00684>.

[68] Elisabetta Farina and others, 'Frequency and Clinical Features of Lewy Body Dementia in Italian Memory Clinics', *Acta Bio-Medica: Atenei Parmensis*, 80.1 (2009), 57–64.

[69] Wei Yue and others, 'The Prevalence of Dementia with Lewy Bodies in a Rural Area of China', *Parkinsonism & Related Disorders*, 29 (2016), 72–77 <https://doi.org/10.1016/j.parkreldis.2016.05.022>.

[70] A. Rongve and others, 'Cognitive Decline in Dementia with Lewy Bodies: A 5-Year Prospective Cohort Study', *BMJ Open*, 6.2 (2016), e010357 <https://doi.org/10.1136/bmjopen-2015-010357>.

[71] Richard A. Goodman and others, 'Prevalence of Dementia Subtypes in United States Medicare Fee-for-Service Beneficiaries, 2011-2013', *Alzheimer's & Dementia: The Journal of the Alzheimer's Association*, 13.1 (2017), 28–37 <https://doi.org/10.1016/j.jalz.2016.04.002>.

[72] Seyed-Mohammad Fereshtehnejad and others, 'Demography, Diagnostics, and Medication in Dementia with Lewy Bodies and Parkinson's Disease with Dementia: Data from the Swedish Dementia Quality Registry (SveDem)', *Neuropsychiatric Disease and Treatment*, 9 (2013), 927–35 <https://doi.org/10.2147/NDT.S45840>.

[73] Annabel Price and others, 'Mortality in Dementia with Lewy Bodies Compared with Alzheimer's Dementia: A Retrospective Naturalistic Cohort Study', *BMJ Open*, 7.11 (2017), e017504 <https://doi.org/10.1136/bmjopen-2017-017504>.

[74] A. Mouton and others, 'Sex Ratio in Dementia with Lewy Bodies Balanced between Alzheimer's Disease and Parkinson's Disease Dementia: A Cross-Sectional

Study', *Alzheimer's Research & Therapy*, 10.1 (2018), 92 <https://doi.org/10.1186/s13195-018-0417-4>.

[75] Andrea M. Kurasz and others, 'Ethnoracial Differences in Lewy Body Diseases with Cognitive Impairment', *Journal of Alzheimer's Disease: JAD*, 77.1 (2020), 165–74 <https://doi.org/10.3233/JAD-200395>.

[76] 'Dementia with Lewy Bodies', *Department of Neurology*, 2020 <https://www.columbianeurology.org/neurology/staywell/dementia-lewy-bodies> [accessed 20 October 2020].

[77] Masaki Takao and others, 'Early-Onset Dementia with Lewy Bodies', *Brain Pathology (Zurich, Switzerland)*, 14.2 (2004), 137–47 <https://doi.org/10.1111/j.1750-3639.2004.tb00046.x>.

[78] 'Lewy Body Dementia Stages, Symptoms & Prognosis', *MedicineNet* <https://www.medicinenet.com/lewy_body_dementia_lbd_symptoms_and_prognosis/views.htm> [accessed 20 October 2020].

[79] Kurt A. Jellinger and Amos D. Korczyn, 'Are Dementia with Lewy Bodies and Parkinson's Disease Dementia the Same Disease?', *BMC Medicine*, 16.1 (2018), 34 <https://doi.org/10.1186/s12916-018-1016-8>.

[80] 'Diagnosis and Treatment of Lewy Body Dementia' <https://www.mentalhelp.net/cognitive-disorders/diagnosis-and-treatment-of-lewy-body-dementia/> [accessed 20 October 2020].

[81] Yuriko Kojima and others, 'Characteristics of Facial Expression Recognition Ability in Patients with Lewy Body Disease', *Environmental Health and Preventive Medicine*, 23.1 (2018), 32 <https://doi.org/10.1186/s12199-018-0723-2>.

[82] James E. Galvin, 'Improving the Clinical Detection of Lewy Body Dementia with the Lewy Body Composite Risk Score', *Alzheimer's & Dementia: Diagnosis, Assessment & Disease Monitoring*, 1.3 (2015), 316–24 <https://doi.org/10.1016/j.dadm.2015.05.004>.

[83] 'Lewy Body Dementia - Symptoms and Causes - Mayo Clinic'.

[84] 'Dementia Symptoms: Illusions, Hallucinations and Delusions' <https://healthblog.uofmhealth.org/brain-health/illusions-hallucinations-and-delusions-how-to-spot-dementia-symptoms> [accessed 18 February 2018].

[85] 'Dementia with Lewy Bodies Symptoms - Six Signs of the Disease | Health | Life & Style | Express.Co.Uk' <https://www.express.co.uk/life-style/health/809643/dementia-lewy-bodies-symptoms-vascular-alzheimers> [accessed 18 February 2018].

[86] 'Lewy Body Dementia' <https://patient.info/health/memory-loss-and-dementia/lewy-body-dementia> [accessed 18 February 2018].

[87] Carolyn Steber, 'Signs Your Brain Fog Is More Serious Than You Might Think', *Bustle* <https://www.bustle.com/p/11-signs-your-brain-might-be-slowing-down-earlier-than-it-should-80166> [accessed 18 February 2018].

[88] 'Lewy Body Dementia - Symptoms and Causes - Mayo Clinic'.

[89] 'How Lewy Body Dementia Contributes to Depression'

<https://www.alzheimers.net/11-21-14-lewy-body-depression-hallucinations/> [accessed 18 February 2018].

[90] 'What Is Lewy Body Dementia?', *WebMD* <https://www.webmd.com/alzheimers/guide/dementia-lewy-bodies> [accessed 18 February 2018].

[91] 'How Lewy Body Dementia Contributes to Depression'.

[92] 'Symptoms | Lewy Body Dementia Association' <https://www.lbda.org/content/symptoms> [accessed 18 February 2018].

[93] 'News You Can Use: Fall Prevention Tips | Lewy Body Dementia Association' <https://www.lbda.org/content/news-you-can-use-fall-prevention-tips> [accessed 18 February 2018].

[94] 'ComparisonofdementiawithLewybidoesto.Pdf' <http://www.cumc.columbia.edu/dept/sergievsky/pdfs/ComparisonofdementiawithLewybidoesto.pdf> [accessed 18 February 2018].

[95] 'Lewy Body Dementia: Information for Patients, Families, and Professionals | Lewy Body Dementia Association' <https://www.lbda.org/content/lewy-body-dementia-information-patients-families-and-professionals> [accessed 18 February 2018].

[96] 'Reduce Dementia-Related Swallowing Problems. Avoid Aspiration. - Lewy Body Dementia' <http://www.lewybodydementia.ca/solve-swallowing-problems-and-avoid-aspiration-in-dementia/> [accessed 18 February 2018].

[97] 'ALZ026-DLB-0116-0118_FEB-2016_WEB.Pdf' <https://www.alzheimersresearchuk.org/wp-content/uploads/2015/02/ALZ026-DLB-0116-0118_FEB-2016_WEB.pdf> [accessed 18 February 2018].

[98] 'Living Well with Lewy Body Dementia and Comorbidities : Dementia and Chest Infections', *Living Well with Lewy Body Dementia and Comorbidities*, 2013 <http://ken-kenc2.blogspot.com/2013/11/dementia-and-chest-infections.html> [accessed 18 February 2018].

[99] 'Lewy Body Dementia - Symptoms and Causes', *Mayo Clinic* <https://www.mayoclinic.org/diseases-conditions/lewy-body-dementia/symptoms-causes/syc-20352025> [accessed 15 November 2019].

[100] 'What Is Lewy Body Dementia?', *National Institute on Aging* <https://www.nia.nih.gov/health/what-lewy-body-dementia> [accessed 15 November 2019].

[101] '10 Things You Should Know about LBD | Lewy Body Dementia Association' <https://www.lbda.org/go/10-things-you-should-know-about-lbd> [accessed 15 November 2019].

[102] 'Dementia with Lewy Bodies - Symptoms', *Nhs.Uk*, 2018 <https://www.nhs.uk/conditions/dementia-with-lewy-bodies/symptoms/> [accessed 15 November 2019].

[103] 'What Is Parkinson's?', *Parkinson's Foundation*, 2015 <https://parkinson.org/understanding-parkinsons/what-is-parkinsons> [accessed 25 April

2019].

[104] 'What Is Parkinson's? | American Parkinson Disease Assoc.', *APDA* <https://www.apdaparkinson.org/what-is-parkinsons/> [accessed 25 April 2019].

[105] 'Ayurveda' <https://www.hopkinsmedicine.org/health/wellness-and-prevention/ayurveda> [accessed 2 December 2020].

[106] Kaviraj Kunja Lal Bhishagratna, *An English Translation of the Sushruta Samhita, Based on Original Sanskrit Text, Vol. 1 of 3: Sutrasthanam* (Place of publication not identified: Forgotten Books, 2018).

[107] 'Sushruta Samhita: The Ancient Treatise on Surgery' <https://www.livehistoryindia.com/snapshort-histories/2017/11/27/sushruta-samhita-the-ancient-treatise-on-surgery> [accessed 2 December 2020].

[108] 'Galen', in *The Stanford Encyclopedia of Philosophy*, ed. by Edward N. Zalta, Winter 2016 (Metaphysics Research Lab, Stanford University, 2016) <https://plato.stanford.edu/archives/win2016/entries/galen/> [accessed 2 December 2020].

[109] 'James Parkinson | Perspectives | Parkinson's Life', *Parkinson's Life*, 2020 <https://parkinsonslife.eu/james-parkinson-the-man-behind-the-shaking-palsy/> [accessed 3 December 2020].

[110] Im Donaldson, 'James Parkinson's Essay on the Shaking Palsy', *The Journal of the Royal College of Physicians of Edinburgh*, 45.1 (2015), 84–86 <https://doi.org/10.4997/JRCPE.2015.118>.

[111] David R. Kumar and others, 'Jean-Martin Charcot: The Father of Neurology', *Clinical Medicine & Research*, 9.1 (2011), 46 <https://doi.org/10.3121/cmr.2009.883>.

[112] 'A Different Sort of Hall-of-Fame: Gehrig, Charcot, and ALS Through History', *ALS Therapy Development Institute* <https://www.als.net/news/a-different-sort-of-hall-of-fame-gehrig-charcot-and-als-through-history/> [accessed 3 December 2020].

[113] Helio A. G. Teive, Renato Puppi Munhoz, and Egberto Reis Barbosa, 'Little-Known Scientific Contributions of J-M Charcot', *Clinics*, 62.3 (2007), 211–14 <https://doi.org/10.1590/S1807-59322007000300003>.

[114] 'Diseases - Charcot-Marie-Tooth Disease (CMT)', *Muscular Dystrophy Association*, 2015 <https://www.mda.org/disease/charcot-marie-tooth> [accessed 3 December 2020].

[115] Christopher G. Goetz, 'Chapter 15 Jean-Martin Charcot and the Anatomo-Clinical Method of Neurology', in *Handbook of Clinical Neurology*, ed. by Michael J. Aminoff, François Boller, and Dick F. Swaab, History of Neurology (Elsevier, 2009), xcv, 203–12 <https://doi.org/10.1016/S0072-9752(08)02115-5>.

[116] 'Parkinson's Disease Statistics', *Parkinson's News Today* <https://parkinsonsnewstoday.com/parkinsons-disease-statistics/> [accessed 25 April 2019].

[117] Amy Reeve, Eve Simcox, and Doug Turnbull, 'Ageing and Parkinson's Disease: Why Is Advancing Age the Biggest Risk Factor?', *Ageing Research Reviews*, 14.100

(2014), 19–30 <https://doi.org/10.1016/j.arr.2014.01.004>.

[118] 'A Look at the Most Common Neurological Disorders', *Classic Rehabilitation, Inc*, 2016 <https://www.classicrehabilitation.com/blog/a-look-at-the-most-common-neurological-disorders/> [accessed 4 December 2020].

[119] 'Statistics', *Parkinson's Foundation* <https://www.parkinson.org/Understanding-Parkinsons/Statistics> [accessed 4 December 2020].

[120] Erum Naqvi, 'Parkinson's Disease Statistics - Parkinson's News Today' <https://parkinsonsnewstoday.com/parkinsons-disease-statistics/> [accessed 4 December 2020].

[121] 'Parkinson's Disease | UCB' <https://www.ucb-canada.ca/en/Patients/Conditions/Parkinson-s-Disease> [accessed 4 December 2020].

[122] Department of Health & Human Services, 'Parkinson's Disease' (Department of Health & Human Services) <https://www.betterhealth.vic.gov.au:443/health/conditionsandtreatments/parkinsons-disease> [accessed 4 December 2020].

[123] R. Norel and others, 'Speech-Based Characterization of Dopamine Replacement Therapy in People with Parkinson's Disease', *Npj Parkinson's Disease*, 6.1 (2020), 1–8 <https://doi.org/10.1038/s41531-020-0113-5>.

[124] Yu Zhang Dagher Kevin Michel-Herve Larcher, Bratislav Misic, and Alain, *English: Substantia Nigra (Shown in Red).*, 2017, Zhang Y, Larcher KM, Misic B, Dagher A. Anatomical and functional organization of the human substantia nigra and its connections. Elife. 2017;6:e26653. Published 2017 Aug 21. https://doi.org/10.7554/eLife.26653.001 <https://commons.wikimedia.org/wiki/File:Substantia_Nigra.png> [accessed 4 December 2020].

[125] 'The Genetic Link to Parkinson's Disease' <https://www.hopkinsmedicine.org/health/conditions-and-diseases/parkinsons-disease/the-genetic-link-to-parkinsons-disease> [accessed 4 December 2020].

[126] 'Young Onset Parkinson's', *Parkinson's Foundation* <https://www.parkinson.org/Understanding-Parkinsons/What-is-Parkinsons/Young-Onset-Parkinsons> [accessed 4 December 2020].

[127] 'Parkinson's Disease - Causes', *Nhs.Uk*, 2018 <https://www.nhs.uk/conditions/parkinsons-disease/causes/> [accessed 4 December 2020].

[128] 'Can Environmental Toxins Cause Parkinson's Disease?' <https://www.hopkinsmedicine.org/health/conditions-and-diseases/parkinsons-disease/can-environmental-toxins-cause-parkinson-disease> [accessed 4 December 2020].

[129] Harvard Health Publishing, 'The Facts about Parkinson's Disease', *Harvard Health* <https://www.health.harvard.edu/diseases-and-conditions/the-facts-about-parkinsons-disease> [accessed 4 December 2020].

[130] Stephen Van Den Eeden and others, 'Incidence of Parkinson's Disease: Variation by Age, Gender, and Race/Ethnicity', *American Journal of Epidemiology*, 157 (2003), 1015–22 <https://doi.org/10.1093/aje/kwg068>.

[131] 'Understanding Parkinson's and Parkinson's Dementia', *Healthline*, 2016 <https://www.healthline.com/health/parkinsons/parkinsons-dementia> [accessed 25 April 2019].

[132] 'Gait Abnormalities', *Stanford Medicine 25* <https://stanfordmedicine25.stanford.edu/the25/gait.html> [accessed 24 April 2019].

[133] 'Dementia' <https://www.who.int/news-room/fact-sheets/detail/dementia> [accessed 13 December 2018].

[134] 'Parkinsons_Disease' <http://www.thepi.org/faq/parkinsons-disease> [accessed 24 April 2019].

[135] 'Non-Movement Symptoms', *Parkinson's Foundation*, 2017 <https://parkinson.org/Understanding-Parkinsons/Non-Movement-Symptoms> [accessed 25 April 2019].

[136] K. Ray Chaudhuri, Daniel G. Healy, and Anthony HV Schapira, 'Non-Motor Symptoms of Parkinson's Disease: Diagnosis and Management', *The Lancet Neurology*, 5.3 (2006), 235–45 <https://doi.org/10.1016/S1474-4422(06)70373-8>.

[137] 'Cognitive Impairment in Parkinson's Disease', *Parkinson's News Today* <https://parkinsonsnewstoday.com/parkinsons-disease-symptoms/non-motor/cognitive-impairment/> [accessed 17 November 2019].

[138] European Parkinson's Disease Association, 'Motor Symptoms' <http://www.epda.eu.com/about-parkinsons/symptoms/motor-symptoms/> [accessed 25 April 2019].

[139] 'Movement Symptoms', *Parkinson's Foundation*, 2017 <https://parkinson.org/Understanding-Parkinsons/Movement-Symptoms> [accessed 25 April 2019].

[140] 'The LBD Spectrum | Lewy Body Dementia Association' <https://www.lbda.org/go/lbd-spectrum> [accessed 25 April 2019].

[141] NeuRA, 'Frontotemporal Dementia', *NeuRA*, 2016 <https://www.neura.edu.au/health/frontotemporal-dementia/> [accessed 15 January 2019].

[142] 'Frontotemporal Dementia', *Memory and Aging Center* <https://memory.ucsf.edu/dementia/ftd> [accessed 28 October 2019].

[143] 'What Are Frontotemporal Disorders?', *National Institute on Aging* <https://www.nia.nih.gov/health/what-are-frontotemporal-disorders> [accessed 28 October 2019].

[144] Daniela Galimberti and Elio Scarpini, 'Genetics of Frontotemporal Lobar Degeneration', *Frontiers in Neurology*, 3 (2012) <https://doi.org/10.3389/fneur.2012.00052>.

[145] T. B. Gislason and others, 'The Prevalence of Frontal Variant Frontotemporal Dementia and the Frontal Lobe Syndrome in a Population Based Sample of 85 Year Olds', *Journal of Neurology, Neurosurgery & Psychiatry*, 74.7 (2003), 867–71 <https://doi.org/10.1136/jnnp.74.7.867>.

[146] Michelle Leahy, 'Fast Facts about Frontotemporal Degeneration', 1.

[147] 'Frontotemporal Dementia' <https://stanfordhealthcare.org/medical-conditions/brain-and-nerves/dementia/types/frontotemporal-dementia.html> [accessed 5 December 2019].

[148] Christer Nilsson and others, 'Age-Related Incidence and Family History in Frontotemporal Dementia: Data from the Swedish Dementia Registry', *PLoS ONE*, 9.4 (2014) <https://doi.org/10.1371/journal.pone.0094901>.

[149] 'Disease Overview', *Association for Frontotemporal Degeneration* <https://www.theaftd.org/understandingftd/ftd-overview> [accessed 18 February 2018].

[150] 'Fast-Facts-Final-11-12.Pdf' <https://www.theaftd.org/wp-content/uploads/2009/05/Fast-Facts-Final-11-12.pdf> [accessed 18 February 2018].

[151] 'Frontotemporal Dementia' <https://www.hopkinsmedicine.org/health/conditions-and-diseases/dementia/frontotemporal-dementia> [accessed 30 October 2019].

[152] 'FAQs', *AFTD* <https://www.theaftd.org/what-is-ftd/faqs/> [accessed 30 October 2019].

[153] 'Frontotemporal Dementia - Health Encyclopedia - University of Rochester Medical Center' <https://www.urmc.rochester.edu/encyclopedia/content.aspx?contenttypeid=134&contentid=77> [accessed 30 October 2019].

[154] 'Posterior Cortical Atrophy', *Wikipedia*, 2018 <https://en.wikipedia.org/w/index.php?title=Posterior_cortical_atrophy&oldid=858211681> [accessed 12 January 2019].

[155] 'Behavioral Variant Frontotemporal Dementia | Memory and Aging Center' <https://memory.ucsf.edu/behavioral-variant-frontotemporal-dementia> [accessed 18 February 2018].

[156] 'Frontotemporal Disorders: Hope Through Research | National Institute of Neurological Disorders and Stroke' <https://www.ninds.nih.gov/Disorders/Patient-Caregiver-Education/Hope-Through-Research/Frontotemporal-Disorders> [accessed 18 February 2018].

[157] 'Frontotemporal Dementia | Johns Hopkins Medicine Health Library' <https://www.hopkinsmedicine.org/healthlibrary/conditions/nervous_system_disorders/frontotemporal_dementia_134,77> [accessed 18 February 2018].

[158] 'Symptoms', *Nhs.Uk* <https://www.nhs.uk/conditions/frontotemporal-dementia/symptoms/> [accessed 18 February 2018].

[159] 'Frontotemporal Dementia' <http://alzheimer.ca/en/Home/About-dementia/Dementias/Frontotemporal-Dementia-and-Pick-s-disease> [accessed 18

February 2018].

[160] 'Dementia Symptoms and Diagnosis - Illnesseses and Conditions | NHS Inform' <https://www.nhsinform.scot/illnesses-and-conditions/brain-nerves-and-spinal-cord/dementia/dementia-symptoms-and-diagnosis/dementia-symptoms-and-diagnosis> [accessed 18 February 2018].

[161] Mette Sagbakken and others, 'Dignity in People with Frontotemporal Dementia and Similar Disorders — a Qualitative Study of the Perspective of Family Caregivers', *BMC Health Services Research*, 17 (2017) <https://doi.org/10.1186/s12913-017-2378-x>.

[162] 'Frontotemporal Dementia | Memory and Aging Center' <https://memory.ucsf.edu/frontotemporal-dementia> [accessed 18 February 2018].

[163] 'Frontotemporal (Frontal Lobe) Dementia: Causes, Symptoms, and Treatments' <https://www.webmd.com/alzheimers/guide/frontotemporal-dementia#1> [accessed 18 February 2018].

[164] 'The Effect of Changed Behaviors of Frontotemporal Dementia on the Stress Level of Informal Caregivers - ProQuest' <https://search.proquest.com/openview/5c9cf3e4aeb9a2bd0689d8de20c82729/1?pq-origsite=gscholar&cbl=18750&diss=y> [accessed 18 February 2018].

[165] 'Frontotemporal Dementia: A Brain Disease That Challenges Definitions of Mental Illness: Page 5 of 5 | Psychiatric Times' <http://www.psychiatrictimes.com/dementia/frontotemporal-dementia-brain-disease-challenges-definitions-mental-illness/page/0/4> [accessed 18 February 2018].

[166] Virginia E. Sturm and others, 'Prosocial Deficits in Behavioral Variant Frontotemporal Dementia Relate to Reward Network Atrophy', *Brain and Behavior*, 7.10 (2017) <https://doi.org/10.1002/brb3.807>.

[167] 'Inflammatory Pathways Link to Obsessive Behaviors in Frontotemporal Dementia - Neuroscience News' <http://neurosciencenews.com/obsessive-behavior-ftd-6490/> [accessed 18 February 2018].

[168] Joyce Fraker and others, 'The Role of the Occupational Therapist in the Management of Neuropsychiatric Symptoms of Dementia in Clinical Settings', *Occupational Therapy In Health Care*, 28.1 (2014), 4–20 <https://doi.org/10.3109/07380577.2013.867468>.

[169] 'Frontotemporal Dementia - an Overview | ScienceDirect Topics' <https://www.sciencedirect.com/topics/neuroscience/frontotemporal-dementia> [accessed 18 February 2018].

[170] 'Frontotemporal Disorders: Hope Through Research | National Institute of Neurological Disorders and Stroke' <https://www.ninds.nih.gov/Disorders/Patient-Caregiver-Education/Hope-Through-Research/Frontotemporal-Disorders> [accessed 18 February 2018].

[171] 'Frontotemporal Dementia: Types, Symptoms, Treatment' <https://www.medicalnewstoday.com/articles/316113.php> [accessed 18 February 2018].

[172] '7 Stages of Frontotemporal Dementia | Exploring Dementia, One Stage at a

Time' <http://exp.stagesofdementia.net/7-stages-of-frontotemporal-dementia/> [accessed 18 February 2018].

[173] 'Frontotemporal Dementia' <http://alzheimer.ca/en/Home/About-dementia/Dementias/Frontotemporal-Dementia-and-Pick-s-disease> [accessed 18 February 2018].

[174] 'Frontotemporal Dementia: Symptoms And Treatment Explained After 40-Year-Old Dies From Disease' <http://www.huffingtonpost.co.uk/entry/frontotemporal-dementia-symptoms-and-treatment-explained_uk_58e21d77e4b0c777f7889878> [accessed 18 February 2018].

[175] 'Pick Disease of the Brain: Causes, Symptoms, and Diagnosis' <https://www.healthline.com/health/picks-disease> [accessed 18 February 2018].

[176] 'Primary Progressive Aphasia - an Overview | ScienceDirect Topics' <https://www.sciencedirect.com/topics/medicine-and-dentistry/primary-progressive-aphasia> [accessed 18 February 2018].

[177] 'PinFTDcare_Newsletter_Spring_2017.Pdf' <https://www.theaftd.org/wp-content/uploads/2017/04/PinFTDcare_Newsletter_Spring_2017.pdf> [accessed 18 February 2018].

[178] 'What Is Pick's Disease, What Are the Symptoms of Frontotemporal Dementia and What Is a Sufferer's Life Expectancy?', *The Sun*, 2017 <https://www.thesun.co.uk/living/2907739/picks-disease-symptoms-frontotemporal-dementia/> [accessed 18 February 2018].

[179] 'Dementia', *American Speech-Language-Hearing Association* <https://www.asha.org/public/speech/disorders/dementia/> [accessed 18 February 2018].

[180] 'Diseases That Cause Dementia | Dementia Care Notes', *Dementia Care Notes, India*, 2010 <https://dementiacarenotes.in/dementia/causes-of-dementia/> [accessed 18 February 2018].

[181] 'Frontotemporal Dementia', 2017 <https://www.centogene.com/science-education/centopedia/factsheets/ngs-panel-genetic-testing-for-frontotemporal-dementia.html> [accessed 18 February 2018].

[182] NeuRA.

[183] NeuRA.

[184] Allan Ajifo, *English: Caricature on the Differences between Right and Left Brain Sides.*, 2014, https://www.flickr.com/photos/125992663@N02/14414603887/ <https://commons.wikimedia.org/wiki/File:Right_brain.jpg> [accessed 18 February 2018].

[185] 'Disease Overview'.

[186] 'Fast-Facts-Final-11-12.Pdf'.

[187] NeuRA.

[188] 'Behavioral Variant Frontotemporal Dementia | Memory and Aging Center'.

[189] '7 Stages of Frontotemporal Dementia | Exploring Dementia, One Stage at a

Time'.

[190] 'Frontotemporal Dementia'.

[191] 'Pick Disease of the Brain: Causes, Symptoms, and Diagnosis'.

[192] 'Primary Progressive Aphasia - an Overview | ScienceDirect Topics'.

[193] 'Diseases That Cause Dementia | Dementia Care Notes'.

[194] 'Frontotemporal Dementia'.

[195] 'Dementia Symptoms and Diagnosis - Illnesseses and Conditions | NHS Inform'.

[196] 'Frontotemporal Dementia: A Brain Disease That Challenges Definitions of Mental Illness: Page 5 of 5 | Psychiatric Times'.

[197] Sturm and others.

[198] Fraker and others.

[199] 'Frontotemporal Dementia: Symptoms And Treatment Explained After 40-Year-Old Dies From Disease'.

[200] 'Frontotemporal Dementia'.

[201] 'Frontotemporal Dementia | Memory and Aging Center'.

[202] 'The Effect of Changed Behaviors of Frontotemporal Dementia on the Stress Level of Informal Caregivers - ProQuest'.

[203] Sagbakken and others.

[204] 'PinFTDcare_Newsletter_Spring_2017.Pdf'.

[205] 'Frontotemporal Dementia - an Overview | ScienceDirect Topics'.

[206] 'Frontotemporal Disorders: Hope Through Research | National Institute of Neurological Disorders and Stroke'.

[207] 'Frontotemporal Dementia | Johns Hopkins Medicine Health Library'.

[208] 'The Penn FTD Center | Behavioral Variant Frontotemporal Dementia (BvFTD)' <https://ftd.med.upenn.edu/about-ftd-related-disorders/what-are-these-conditions/behavioral-variant-frontotemporal-dementia-bvftd> [accessed 14 January 2019].

[209] 'Behavioral Variant Frontotemporal Dementia', *Memory and Aging Center* <https://memory.ucsf.edu/behavioral-variant-frontotemporal-dementia> [accessed 14 January 2019].

[210] 'Progressive Supranuclear Palsy Fact Sheet | National Institute of Neurological Disorders and Stroke' <https://www.ninds.nih.gov/disorders/patient-caregiver-education/fact-sheets/progressive-supranuclear-palsy-fact-sheet> [accessed 4 December 2019].

[211] 'Progressive Supranuclear Palsy (PSP) | Asceneuron' <https://www.asceneuron.com/progressive-supranuclear-palsy-psp> [accessed 5

December 2019].

[212] 'Parkinson-Plus Syndromes: Clues to Diagnosis, Multiple System Atrophy, Progressive Supranuclear Palsy', 2019 <https://emedicine.medscape.com/article/1154074-overview#a3> [accessed 5 December 2019].

[213] 'Progressive Supranuclear Palsy Fact Sheet | National Institute of Neurological Disorders and Stroke'.

[214] R. W. Shin and others, 'Hydrated Autoclave Pretreatment Enhances Tau Immunoreactivity in Formalin-Fixed Normal and Alzheimer's Disease Brain Tissues', *Laboratory Investigation; a Journal of Technical Methods and Pathology*, 64.5 (1991), 693–702.

[215] Nicolas Sergeant, André Delacourte, and Luc Buée, 'Tau Protein as a Differential Biomarker of Tauopathies', *Biochimica et Biophysica Acta (BBA) - Molecular Basis of Disease*, The Biology and Pathobiology of Tau, 1739.2 (2005), 179–97 <https://doi.org/10.1016/j.bbadis.2004.06.020>.

[216] 'Progressive Supranuclear Palsy (PSP) | Asceneuron'.

[217] 'Progressive Supranuclear Palsy - Symptoms', *Nhs.Uk*, 2018 <https://www.nhs.uk/conditions/progressive-supranuclear-palsy-psp/symptoms/> [accessed 7 December 2019].

[218] 'Progressive Supranuclear Palsy Fact Sheet | National Institute of Neurological Disorders and Stroke' <https://www.ninds.nih.gov/disorders/patient-caregiver-education/fact-sheets/progressive-supranuclear-palsy-fact-sheet> [accessed 7 December 2019].

[219] 'Primary Progressive Aphasia' <https://www.brain.northwestern.edu/dementia/ppa/index.html> [accessed 25 October 2019].

[220] INSERM US14-- ALL RIGHTS RESERVED, 'Orphanet: Primary Progressive Aphasia' <https://www.orpha.net/consor/cgi-bin/OC_Exp.php?lng=en&Expert=95432> [accessed 28 April 2019].

[221] 'Primary Progressive Aphasia', *National Aphasia Association* <https://www.aphasia.org/aphasia-resources/primary-progressive-aphasia/> [accessed 15 January 2019].

[222] Genetics Home Reference, 'TARDBP Gene', *Genetics Home Reference* <https://ghr.nlm.nih.gov/gene/TARDBP> [accessed 6 May 2019].

[223] Edward B. Lee and others, 'Expansion of the Classification of FTLD-TDP: Distinct Pathology Associated with Rapidly Progressive Frontotemporal Degeneration', *Acta Neuropathologica*, 134.1 (2017), 65–78 <https://doi.org/10.1007/s00401-017-1679-9>.

[224] Neuroscience News, 'When Is Alzheimer's Not Alzheimer's? Researchers Characterize a Different Form of Dementia', *Neuroscience News*, 2019 <https://neurosciencenews.com/dementia-tdp-43-late-12090/> [accessed 7 May 2019].

[225] V. M. Lee, M. Goedert, and J. Q. Trojanowski, 'Neurodegenerative Tauopathies', *Annual Review of Neuroscience*, 24 (2001), 1121–59 <https://doi.org/10.1146/annurev.neuro.24.1.1121>.

[226] 'Frontotemporal Dementias' <http://neuropathology-web.org/chapter9/chapter9cFTD.html> [accessed 27 October 2019].

[227] 'The Penn FTD Center | Nonfluent/Agrammatic Primary Progressive Aphasia (Progressive Non-Fluent Aphasia)' <https://ftd.med.upenn.edu/about-ftd-related-disorders/what-are-these-conditions/progressive-language/progressive-nonfluent-aphasia-pna> [accessed 27 April 2019].

[228] Murray Grossman, 'THE NON-FLUENT/AGRAMMATIC VARIANT OF PRIMARY PROGRESSIVE APHASIA', *Lancet Neurology*, 11.6 (2012), 545–55 <https://doi.org/10.1016/S1474-4422(12)70099-6>.

[229] 'Nonfluent Variant Primary Progressive Aphasia', *Memory and Aging Center* <https://memory.ucsf.edu/dementia/primary-progressive-aphasia/nonfluent-variant-primary-progressive-aphasia> [accessed 5 December 2019].

[230] Serena Amici and others, 'An Overview on Primary Progressive Aphasia and Its Variants', *Behavioural Neurology*, 17.2 (2006), 77–87.

[231] Maxime Montembeault and others, 'Clinical, Anatomical, and Pathological Features in the Three Variants of Primary Progressive Aphasia: A Review', *Frontiers in Neurology*, 9 (2018) <https://doi.org/10.3389/fneur.2018.00692>.

[232] Grossman, 'THE NON-FLUENT/AGRAMMATIC VARIANT OF PRIMARY PROGRESSIVE APHASIA'.

[233] Bruce L. Miller, *The Clinical Syndrome of SvPPA* (Oxford University Press) <http://oxfordmedicine.com/view/10.1093/med/9780195380491.001.0001/med-9780195380491-chapter-3> [accessed 27 April 2019].

[234] Leonardo Iaccarino and others, 'The Semantic Variant of Primary Progressive Aphasia: Clinical and Neuroimaging Evidence in Single Subjects', *PLoS ONE*, 10.3 (2015) <https://doi.org/10.1371/journal.pone.0120197>.

[235] 'Patterns of Temporal Lobe Atrophy in Semantic Dementia and Alzheimer's Disease - Chan - 2001 - Annals of Neurology - Wiley Online Library' <https://onlinelibrary.wiley.com/doi/abs/10.1002/ana.92> [accessed 27 April 2019].

[236] Grossman, 'THE NON-FLUENT/AGRAMMATIC VARIANT OF PRIMARY PROGRESSIVE APHASIA'.

[237] 'Semantic Variant Primary Progressive Aphasia', *Memory and Aging Center* <https://memory.ucsf.edu/dementia/primary-progressive-aphasia/semantic-variant-primary-progressive-aphasia> [accessed 6 December 2019].

[238] 'The Penn FTD Center | Semantic Variant Primary Progressive Aphasia

(Semantic Dementia)' <https://ftd.med.upenn.edu/about-ftd-related-disorders/what-are-these-conditions/progressive-language/semantic-variant-primary-progressive-aphasia-svppa> [accessed 29 April 2019].

[239] Murray Grossman, 'Primary Progressive Aphasia: Clinicopathological Correlations', *Nature Reviews. Neurology*, 6.2 (2010), 88–97 <https://doi.org/10.1038/nrneurol.2009.216>.

[240] Murray Grossman, 'THE NON-FLUENT/AGRAMMATIC VARIANT OF PRIMARY PROGRESSIVE APHASIA', *Lancet Neurology*, 11.6 (2012), 545–55 <https://doi.org/10.1016/S1474-4422(12)70099-6>.

[241] M.L. Gorno-Tempini and others, 'Classification of Primary Progressive Aphasia and Its Variants', *Neurology*, 76.11 (2011), 1006–14 <https://doi.org/10.1212/WNL.0b013e31821103e6>.

[242] 'Vascular Dementia: Background, Pathophysiology, Epidemiology', 2019 <https://emedicine.medscape.com/article/292105-overview> [accessed 14 June 2019].

[243] 'Updates to DSM-5 Criteria & Text' <https://www.psychiatry.org/psychiatrists/practice/dsm/updates-to-dsm-5//updates-to-dsm-5-criteria-text> [accessed 14 June 2019].

[244] Kurt A. Jellinger, 'The Enigma of Mixed Dementia', *Alzheimer's & Dementia: The Journal of the Alzheimer's Association*, 3.1 (2007), 40–53 <https://doi.org/10.1016/j.jalz.2006.09.002>.

[245] 'Vascular Dementia and Vascular Cognitive Impairment: A Resource List', *National Institute on Aging* <https://www.nia.nih.gov/health/vascular-dementia-and-vascular-cognitive-impairment-resource-list> [accessed 16 June 2019].

[246] 'Vascular Dementia | Memory and Aging Center' <https://memory.ucsf.edu/vascular-dementia> [accessed 18 February 2018].

[247] Hollie Richardson, 'Vascular Dementia', *Alzheimer's Society* <https://www.alzheimers.org.uk/info/20007/types_of_dementia/5/vascular_dementia/8> [accessed 18 February 2018].

[248] 'Different Types of Dementia', *Dementia Statistics Hub* <https://www.dementiastatistics.org/statistics/different-types-of-dementia/> [accessed 26 December 2018].

[249] Gustavo C Román and others, 'Subcortical Ischaemic Vascular Dementia', *The Lancet Neurology*, 1.7 (2002), 426–36 <https://doi.org/10.1016/S1474-4422(02)00190-4>.

[250] 'Causes', *Nhs.Uk*, 2018 <https://www.nhs.uk/conditions/vascular-dementia/causes/> [accessed 16 June 2019].

[251] Milija D. Mijajlović and others, 'Post-Stroke Dementia – a Comprehensive Review', *BMC Medicine*, 15 (2017) <https://doi.org/10.1186/s12916-017-0779-7>.

[252] Daniel Gorman, 'Post Stroke Dementia: Diagnosis & Intervention', 43.

[253] 'Brain | Oxford Academic', *OUP Academic* <https://academic.oup.com/brain>

[accessed 16 June 2019].

[254] <img src='//sgec stanford edu/content/dam/sm-news/images/2015/08/goldman-bruce-90 jpg img 620 high png' alt='Bruce Goldman'> By Bruce Goldman Bruce Goldman is a science writer for the medical school's Office of Communication & Public Affairs Email him at goldmanb@stanford.edu, 'Immune Profile Two Days after Stroke Predicts Dementia a Year Later', *News Center* <http://med.stanford.edu/news/all-news/2019/03/immune-profile-two-days-after-stroke-predicts-dementia-a-year-later.html> [accessed 16 June 2019].

[255] Jia-Hao Sun, Lan Tan, and Jin-Tai Yu, 'Post-Stroke Cognitive Impairment: Epidemiology, Mechanisms and Management', *Annals of Translational Medicine*, 2.8 (2014) <https://doi.org/10.3978/j.issn.2305-5839.2014.08.05>.

[256] Elisabeth Höwler, '[Biography and dementia. Origin of challenging behavior in patients with multi-infarct dementia or senile dementia of the Alzheimer type in long term care with reference the biographical level]', *Pflege Zeitschrift*, 64.10 (2011), 612–15.

[257] 'Multi-Infarct Dementia: Care Instructions' <https://myhealth.alberta.ca:443/Health/aftercareinformation/pages/conditions.aspx?hwid=tw12306> [accessed 16 June 2019].

[258] 'Multi-Infarct Dementia Information Page | National Institute of Neurological Disorders and Stroke' <https://www.ninds.nih.gov/Disorders/All-Disorders/Multi-Infarct-Dementia-Information-Page> [accessed 15 June 2019].

[259] 'Articles | Dementia Research | University of Exeter' <http://www.exeter.ac.uk/dementia/news/articles/strokedoublesdementiarisk.html> [accessed 15 June 2019].

[260] 'University of Exeter' <http://www.exeter.ac.uk/news/archive/2018/august/title_678124_en.html> [accessed 15 June 2019].

[261] 'Binswanger Encephalopathy - an Overview | ScienceDirect Topics' <https://www.sciencedirect.com/topics/medicine-and-dentistry/binswanger-encephalopathy> [accessed 14 June 2019].

[262] Eliasz Engelhardt and Lea T. Grinberg, 'Alzheimer and Vascular Brain Diseases: Focal and Diffuse Subforms', *Dementia & Neuropsychologia*, 9.3 (2015), 306–10 <https://doi.org/10.1590/1980-57642015DN93000015>.

[263] 'Binswanger's Disease Information Page | National Institute of Neurological Disorders and Stroke' <https://www.ninds.nih.gov/Disorders/All-Disorders/Binswangers-Disease-Information-Page> [accessed 14 June 2019].

[264] V Babikian and A H Ropper, 'Binswanger's Disease: A Review.', *Stroke*, 18.1 (1987), 2–12 <https://doi.org/10.1161/01.STR.18.1.2>.

[265] 'Binswanger Encephalopathy - an Overview | ScienceDirect Topics'.

[266] Timo Erkinjuntti, 'Subcortical Ischemic Vascular Disease and Dementia', *International Psychogeriatrics*, 15.S1 (2003), 23–26 <https://doi.org/10.1017/S1041610203008925>.

[267] 'Subcortical Vascular Dementia', *Cleveland Clinic* <https://my.clevelandclinic.org/health/diseases/17520-subcortical-vascular-dementia> [accessed 13 June 2019].

[268] J. L. Cummings and D. F. Benson, 'Subcortical Dementia. Review of an Emerging Concept', *Archives of Neurology*, 41.8 (1984), 874–79 <https://doi.org/10.1001/archneur.1984.04050190080019>.

[269] 'What Is Alzheimer's Disease?', *National Institute on Aging* <https://www.nia.nih.gov/health/what-alzheimers-disease> [accessed 28 November 2018].

[270] '2017-Facts-and-Figures.Pdf' <https://www.alz.org/documents_custom/2017-facts-and-figures.pdf> [accessed 18 February 2018].

[271] 'Alzheimer's Society of America » Alzheimer's Disease' <http://alzheimerssocietyofamerica.org/dementia/alzheimers-disease/> [accessed 18 February 2018].

[272] 'What Is Alzheimer's?', *Alzheimer's Disease and Dementia* <https://alz.org/alzheimers-dementia/what-is-alzheimers> [accessed 28 November 2018].

[273] 'Alzheimer's Disease - Symptoms and Causes', *Mayo Clinic* <http://www.mayoclinic.org/diseases-conditions/alzheimers-disease/symptoms-causes/syc-20350447> [accessed 29 November 2018].

[274] 'Alzheimer's Disease', *Alzheimer's Society* <https://www.alzheimers.org.uk/about-dementia/types-dementia/alzheimers-disease> [accessed 28 November 2018].

[275] <img src='//sgec stanford edu/content/dam/sm-profiles/profileBGoldmanM jpg img 620 high png' alt='Bruce Goldman'> By Bruce Goldman Bruce Goldman is a science writer for the medical school's Office of Communication & Public Affairs, 'Scientists Reveal How Beta-Amyloid May Cause Alzheimer's', *News Center* <http://med.stanford.edu/news/all-news/2013/09/scientists-reveal-how-beta-amyloid-may-cause-alzheimers.html> [accessed 12 December 2018].

[276] 'What Is Alzheimer's Disease?', *National Institute on Aging* <https://www.nia.nih.gov/health/what-alzheimers-disease> [accessed 12 December 2018].

[277] Robin Seaton Jefferson, 'UT Southwestern Medical Center Researchers Discover Alzheimer's Vaccine, Hope To Test In Humans Soon', *Forbes* <https://www.forbes.com/sites/robinseatonjefferson/2018/11/23/ut-researchers-discover-alzheimers-vaccine-hope-to-test-in-humans-soon/> [accessed 12 December 2018].

[278] Roger N. Rosenberg, Min Fu, and Doris Lambracht-Washington, 'Active Full-Length DNA Aβ42 Immunization in 3xTg-AD Mice Reduces Not Only Amyloid Deposition but Also Tau Pathology', *Alzheimer's Research & Therapy*, 10.1 (2018), 115 <https://doi.org/10.1186/s13195-018-0441-4>.

[279] 'Symptoms of Early Onset Dementia' <https://www.hopkinsmedicine.org/healthlibrary/conditions/adult/nervous_system_disorders/early-onset_alzheimer_disease_134,63> [accessed 29 November 2018].

[280] 'Younger/Early Onset', *Alzheimer's Disease and Dementia*

<https://alz.org/alzheimers-dementia/what-is-alzheimers/younger-early-onset> [accessed 12 December 2018].

[281] 'Symptoms of Early Onset Dementia' <https://www.hopkinsmedicine.org/healthlibrary/conditions/adult/nervous_system_disorders/early-onset_alzheimer_disease_134,63> [accessed 12 December 2018].

[282] The Editors, 'What Is Alzheimer's Disease? A Visual Primer', *Scientific American* <https://www.scientificamerican.com/article/what-is-alzheimers-disease-visual-primer/> [accessed 13 December 2018].

[283] 'Number of Alzheimer's Deaths Found to Be Underreported', *National Institute on Aging* <https://www.nia.nih.gov/news/number-alzheimers-deaths-found-be-underreported> [accessed 13 December 2018].

[284] 'Prevalence of Alzheimer's', 1.

[285] '2018 Alzheimer's Disease Facts and Figures', *Alzheimer's & Dementia: The Journal of the Alzheimer's Association*, 14.3 (2018), 367–429 <https://doi.org/10.1016/j.jalz.2018.02.001>.

[286] CDC, 'Deaths from Alzheimer's Disease', *Centers for Disease Control and Prevention*, 2017 <https://www.cdc.gov/features/alzheimers-disease-deaths/index.html> [accessed 13 December 2018].

[287] 'Alzheimer's Disease: Facts & Figures', *BrightFocus Foundation*, 2015 <https://www.brightfocus.org/alzheimers/article/alzheimers-disease-facts-figures> [accessed 30 November 2018].

[288] 'Latest Estimate: One New Case of Dementia Every 3.2 Seconds Archives', *Dementia Alliance International* <https://www.dementiaallianceinternational.org/tag/latest-estimate-one-new-case-of-dementia-every-3-2-seconds/> [accessed 13 December 2018].

[289] 'Dementia'.

[290] 'Alzheimer's Disease Facts and Figures'.

[291] 'World Alzheimer Report 2018 - The State of the Art of Dementia Research: New Frontiers', *NEW FRONTIERS*, 48.

[292] 'Causes of Death', *Our World in Data* <https://ourworldindata.org/causes-of-death> [accessed 13 December 2018].

[293] 'Dementia Risk Factors', *Queensland Brain Institute*, 2017 <https://qbi.uq.edu.au/dementia/dementia-risk-factors> [accessed 13 December 2018].

[294] 'How Does Alzheimer's Affect Women and Men Differently? | Cognitive Vitality | Alzheimer's Drug Discovery Foundation' <https://www.alzdiscovery.org/cognitive-vitality/blog/how-does-alzheimers-affect-women-and-men-differently> [accessed 13 December 2018].

[295] E Willetta St, 'As Our Country Ages, the Number of People Touched by Alzheimer's Only Continues to Increase. Already, More than a Third of the U.S. Adult Population Has Some Personal Connection to the Disease, through a Spouse, Family Member or Other Blood Relative.', 2.

[296] 'How Alzheimer's Could Be Type 2 Diabetes', *Alzheimers.Net*, 2016 <https://www.alzheimers.net/2015-10-14/how-alzheimers-could-be-type-2-diabetes/> [accessed 13 December 2018].

[297] 'Facts about the Connection between Down Syndrome and Alzheimer's Disease', *Global Down Syndrome Foundation*, 2012 <https://www.globaldownsyndrome.org/about-down-syndrome/facts-about-down-syndrome/facts-about-the-connection-between-down-syndrome-and-alzheimers-disease/> [accessed 13 December 2018].

[298] 'Higher Blood Pressure at Midlife Increases Your Risk for Dementia' <https://www.alzheimers.net/higher-blood-pressure-increases-your-risk-for-dementia/> [accessed 13 December 2018].

[299] J. Carson Smith and others, 'Physical Activity and Brain Function in Older Adults at Increased Risk for Alzheimer's Disease', *Brain Sciences*, 3.1 (2013), 54–83 <https://doi.org/10.3390/brainsci3010054>.

[300] 'Obesity: A Risk Factor for Alzheimer's', *Health Essentials from Cleveland Clinic*, 2013 <https://health.clevelandclinic.org/obesity-a-risk-factor-for-alzheimers/> [accessed 13 December 2018].

[301] 'Nine Lifestyle Factors May Lower Your Alzheimer's Risk | Cognitive Vitality | Alzheimer's Drug Discovery Foundation' <https://www.alzdiscovery.org/cognitive-vitality/blog/nine-lifestyle-factors-may-lower-your-alzheimers-risk> [accessed 13 December 2018].

[302] 'Geoba.Se: Gazetteer - United States - 2019 - Statistics and Rankings' <http://www.geoba.se/country.php?cc=US&year=2019> [accessed 28 November 2018].

[303] Adrian O'Dowd, 'Dementia Is Now Leading Cause of Death in Women in England', *BMJ*, 358 (2017), j3445 <https://doi.org/10.1136/bmj.j3445>.

[304] 'Deaths Registered in England and Wales (Series DR) - Office for National Statistics' <https://www.ons.gov.uk/peoplepopulationandcommunity/birthsdeathsandmarriages/deaths/bulletins/deathsregisteredinenglandandwalesseriesdr/2016> [accessed 13 December 2018].

[305] 'Women and Alzheimer's Disease: A Global Epidemic', *NWHN*, 2015 <https://www.nwhn.org/women-and-alzheimers-disease-a-global-epidemic/> [accessed 13 December 2018].

[306] 'WHO | Top 10 Causes of Death', *WHO* <https://doi.org//entity/gho/mortality_burden_disease/causes_death/top_10/en/index.html>.

[307] Yan Zhou and others, 'African Americans Are Less Likely to Enroll in Preclinical Alzheimer's Disease Clinical Trials', *Alzheimer's & Dementia: Translational Research & Clinical Interventions*, 3.1 (2017), 57–64 <https://doi.org/10.1016/j.trci.2016.09.004>.

[308] 'Likelihood of Dementia Higher among Black Ethnic Groups', *EurekAlert!* <https://www.eurekalert.org/pub_releases/2018-08/ucl-lod080618.php> [accessed 13

December 2018].

[309] 'Likelihood of Dementia Higher among Black Ethnic Groups' <https://medicalxpress.com/news/2018-08-likelihood-dementia-higher-black-ethnic.html> [accessed 13 December 2018].

[310] 'Dementia Rates Higher among Black People, New Study Finds', *The Independent*, 2018 <https://www.independent.co.uk/news/health/dementia-black-white-asian-ethnicity-alzheimers-disease-memory-a8481786.html> [accessed 13 December 2018].

[311] 'New Alzheimer's Association Report Reveals Sharp Increases in Alzheimer's Prevalence, Deaths and Cos', *Alzheimer's Disease and Dementia* <https://alz.org/news/2018/new_alzheimer_s_association_report_reveals_sharp_i> [accessed 13 December 2018].

[312] Bruce Japsen, 'Alzheimer's Costs Reach $277 Billion', *Forbes* <https://www.forbes.com/sites/brucejapsen/2018/03/20/alzheimers-costs-reach-277-billion/> [accessed 29 November 2018].

[313] Jianping Jia and others, 'The Cost of Alzheimer's Disease in China and Re-Estimation of Costs Worldwide', *Alzheimer's & Dementia: The Journal of the Alzheimer's Association*, 14.4 (2018), 483–91 <https://doi.org/10.1016/j.jalz.2017.12.006>.

[314] '2018 Alzheimer's Facts & Figures' <http://www.alzheimersweekly.com/2018/03/2018-alzheimers-facts-figures.html> [accessed 13 December 2018].

[315] 'Alzheimer's Disease Consists of Three Distinct Subtypes, According to UCLA Study', *UCLA* <http://newsroom.ucla.edu/releases/alzheimers-disease-consists-of-three-distinct-subtypes-according-to-ucla-study> [accessed 12 November 2019].

[316] 'Leading The Charge: Expanding Collaborative, Cross-Disciplinary Research for the Prevention, Treatment, and Care of Dementia — Bypass Budget FY22', *National Institute on Aging* <http://www.nia.nih.gov/about/leading-charge-expanding-collaborative-cross-disciplinary-research-prevention-treatment> [accessed 21 March 2022].

[317] Liesi E. Hebert and others, 'Alzheimer Disease in the United States (2010–2050) Estimated Using the 2010 Census', *Neurology*, 80.19 (2013), 1778–83 <https://doi.org/10.1212/WNL.0b013e31828726f5>.

[318] 'The 50 US States Ranked By Population', *WorldAtlas* <https://www.worldatlas.com/articles/us-states-by-population.html> [accessed 30 November 2018].

[319] 'Dementia Statistics – U.S. & Worldwide Stats', *BrainTest*, 2015 <https://braintest.com/dementia-stats-u-s-worldwide/> [accessed 1 December 2018].

[320] 'Americans With Alzheimer's Now Number 5.7 Million' <https://www.forbes.com/sites/nextavenue/2018/03/25/americans-with-alzheimers-now-number-5-7-million/#70db8124b627> [accessed 1 December 2018].

[321] 'Fiscal Year 2019 Alzheimer's Research Funding', 1.

[322] 'Alzheimer's Disease'.

[323] 'Facts and Figures', *Alzheimer's Disease and Dementia* <https://alz.org/alzheimers-dementia/facts-figures> [accessed 30 November 2018].

[324] 'WHO | Dementia Cases Set to Triple by 2050 but Still Largely Ignored', *WHO* <https://www.who.int/mediacentre/news/releases/2012/dementia_20120411/en/> [accessed 30 November 2018].

[325] 'Ten Countries with the Highest Population in the World' <https://www.internetworldstats.com/stats8.htm> [accessed 30 November 2018].

[326] 'How Many Countries Are There in the World? (2018) - Total & List | Worldometers' <http://www.worldometers.info/geography/how-many-countries-are-there-in-the-world/> [accessed 30 November 2018].

[327] 'When Alzheimer's Symptoms Start before Age 65', *Mayo Clinic* <https://www.mayoclinic.org/diseases-conditions/alzheimers-disease/in-depth/alzheimers/art-20048356> [accessed 2 December 2019].

[328] Genetics Home Reference, 'What Is a Chromosome?', *Genetics Home Reference* <https://ghr.nlm.nih.gov/primer/basics/chromosome> [accessed 2 December 2019].

[329] 'What Are Chromosomes?' <https://www.healio.com/hematology-oncology/learn-genomics/genomics-primer/what-are-chromosomes> [accessed 2 December 2019].

[330] File:Chromosome-es svg: KES47, *English: Graphic Decomposition of a Chromosome (Found in the Cell Nucleus), to the Bases Pair of the DNA.*, 2010, File:Chromosome-es.svg <https://commons.wikimedia.org/wiki/File:Chromosome_en.svg> [accessed 2 December 2019].

[331] Genetics Home Reference, 'Chromosome 1', *Genetics Home Reference* <https://ghr.nlm.nih.gov/chromosome/1> [accessed 2 December 2019].

[332] Genetics Home Reference, 'PSEN2 Gene', *Genetics Home Reference* <https://ghr.nlm.nih.gov/gene/PSEN2> [accessed 2 December 2019].

[333] 'Chromosome 21 - an Overview | ScienceDirect Topics' <https://www.sciencedirect.com/topics/neuroscience/chromosome-21> [accessed 3 December 2019].

[334] National Human Genome Research Institute, *English: Human Male Karyotype after G-Banding. Chromosome 21 Highlighted*, 2015, File:Human male karyotype high resolution.jpg <https://commons.wikimedia.org/wiki/File:Human_male_karyotype_high_resolution_-_Chromosome_21.png> [accessed 1 December 2019].

[335] Byron Creese and others, 'AN EVALUATION OF PREDICTORS AND COGNITIVE DECLINE ASSOCIATED WITH PERSISTENT AND TRANSIENT PSYCHOTIC SYMPTOMS IN ALZHEIMER'S DISEASE', *Alzheimer's & Dementia: The Journal of the Alzheimer's Association*, 13.7 (2017), P367 <https://doi.org/10.1016/j.jalz.2017.06.315>.

[336] Ilona Hallikainen and others, 'The Progression of Neuropsychiatric Symptoms in Alzheimer's Disease During a Five-Year Follow-Up: Kuopio ALSOVA Study', *Journal of Alzheimer's Disease*, 61.4 (2018), 1367–76 <https://doi.org/10.3233/JAD-170697>.

[337] Sheridan T. Read, Christine Toye, and Dianne Wynaden, 'Experiences and Expectations of Living with Dementia: A Qualitative Study', *Collegian*, 24.5 (2017), 427–32 <https://doi.org/10.1016/j.colegn.2016.09.003>.

[338] undefined, 'How to Tell Alzheimer's Disease from "normal" Memory Loss', *Cleveland.Com*, 2011 <http://www.cleveland.com/healthfit/index.ssf/2011/04/how_to_tell_alzheimers_disease.html> [accessed 14 December 2018].

[339] 'When a Person with Alzheimer's Rummages and Hides Things', *National Institute on Aging* <https://www.nia.nih.gov/health/when-person-alzheimers-rummages-and-hides-things> [accessed 14 December 2018].

[340] Katherine Kam, 'Memory Loss With Alzheimer's Disease: What to Expect', *WebMD* <https://www.webmd.com/alzheimers/features/dealing-with-alzheimers-disease-memory-loss> [accessed 14 December 2018].

[341] Tara E. Tracy and Li Gan, 'Acetylated Tau in Alzheimer's Disease: An Instigator of Synaptic Dysfunction Underlying Memory Loss', *BioEssays*, 39.4 (2017), n/a-n/a <https://doi.org/10.1002/bies.201600224>.

[342] 'Brain Tour', *Alzheimer's Disease and Dementia* <https://alz.org/alzheimers-dementia/what-is-alzheimers/brain_tour> [accessed 14 December 2018].

[343] Holger Jahn, 'Memory Loss in Alzheimer's Disease', *Dialogues in Clinical Neuroscience*, 15.4 (2013), 445–54 <https://www.ncbi.nlm.nih.gov/pmc/articles/PMC3898682/> [accessed 14 December 2018].

[344] 'How Do People Experience Memory Loss?', *Alzheimer's Society* <https://www.alzheimers.org.uk/about-dementia/symptoms-and-diagnosis/symptoms/memory-loss-in-dementia> [accessed 14 December 2018].

[345] 'Memory Loss: When to Seek Help', *Mayo Clinic* <https://www.mayoclinic.org/diseases-conditions/alzheimers-disease/in-depth/memory-loss/art-20046326> [accessed 14 December 2018].

[346] 'Normal Aging vs Dementia | Alzheimer Society of Canada' <http://alzheimer.ca/en/Home/About-dementia/What-is-dementia/Normal-aging-vs-dementia> [accessed 14 December 2018].

[347] 'Alzheimer's Disease', *Memory and Aging Center* <https://memory.ucsf.edu/alzheimer-disease> [accessed 14 December 2018].

[348] Nancy L. Mace and Peter V. Rabins, *The 36-Hour Day: A Family Guide to Caring for People Who Have Alzheimer Disease, Other Dementias, and Memory Loss* (JHU Press, 2017).

[349] 'When Alzheimer's Turns Violent' <http://www.cnn.com/2011/HEALTH/03/30/alzheimers.violence.caregiving/index.html>

[accessed 14 December 2018].

[350] 'Alzheimer's: 25 Signs Never to Ignore' <https://www.cbsnews.com/pictures/alzheimers-25-signs-never-to-ignore/> [accessed 14 December 2018].

[351] 'Treatments for Behavior', *Alzheimer's Disease and Dementia* <https://alz.org/alzheimers-dementia/treatments/treatments-for-behavior> [accessed 14 December 2018].

[352] 'LATE Dementia Is a New Type of Brain Disease That Mimics Alzheimer's', *Being Patient*, 2019 <https://www.beingpatient.com/late-dementia/> [accessed 6 May 2019].

[353] Sarah Knapton, 'Hundreds of Thousands with Alzheimer's Are Probably Suffering from Late Disease, Scientists Say', *The Telegraph*, 30 April 2019 <https://www.telegraph.co.uk/science/2019/04/30/hundreds-thousands-alzheimers-probably-suffering-late-disease/> [accessed 5 May 2019].

[354] 'Researchers Define Alzheimer's-like Brain Disorder', *EurekAlert!* <https://eurekalert.org/pub_releases/2019-04/rumc-rda043019.php> [accessed 3 May 2019].

[355] 'What Happens to the Brain in Alzheimer's Disease?', *National Institute on Aging* <https://www.nia.nih.gov/health/what-happens-brain-alzheimers-disease> [accessed 6 May 2019].

[356] 'Stages of Alzheimer's', *Alzheimer's Disease and Dementia* <https://alz.org/alzheimers-dementia/stages> [accessed 6 May 2019].

[357] Peter T. Nelson and others, 'Limbic-Predominant Age-Related TDP-43 Encephalopathy (LATE): Consensus Working Group Report', *Brain* <https://doi.org/10.1093/brain/awz099>.

[358] 'New Dementia Classification for Disease with Alzheimer's like Symptoms', *Alzheimer's Research UK*, 2019 <https://www.alzheimersresearchuk.org/new-dementia-classification-for-disease-with-alzheimers-like-symptoms/> [accessed 6 May 2019].

[359] Allan Adamson, 'New Form Of Dementia LATE Can Be Mistaken As Alzheimer's Disease', *Tech Times*, 2019 <https://www.techtimes.com/articles/242662/20190430/newly-recognized-form-of-dementia-is-sometimes-mistaken-as-alzheimers-how-to-recognize-this-brain-disorder.htm> [accessed 6 May 2019].

[360] 'Guidelines Proposed for Newly Defined Alzheimer's-like Brain Disorder', *National Institute on Aging* <https://www.nia.nih.gov/news/guidelines-proposed-newly-defined-alzheimers-brain-disorder> [accessed 6 May 2019].

[361] 'Nina SILVERBERG', *National Institute on Aging* <https://www.nia.nih.gov/about/staff/silverberg-nina> [accessed 6 May 2019].

[362] 'Richard HODES', *National Institute on Aging* <https://www.nia.nih.gov/about/staff/hodes-richard> [accessed 6 May 2019].

[363] Nina Silverberg, 'The Alzheimer's Disease Centers Program: Updates', 28.

[364] 'Researchers Define Alzheimer's-like Brain Disorder: LATE Symptoms Resembles Alzheimer's Disease but Has Different Cause', *ScienceDaily* <https://www.sciencedaily.com/releases/2019/04/190430121800.htm> [accessed 1 May 2019].

[365] John Gibbs, 'New Type of Dementia Is "100 Times More Common" than ALS', *Medicine News Line*, 2019 <https://medkit.info/2019/05/01/new-type-of-dementia-is-100-times-more-common-than-als/> [accessed 6 May 2019].

[366] 'Not Too Late to Focus on LATE, an Overlooked Brain Disease', *GEN - Genetic Engineering and Biotechnology News*, 2019 <https://www.genengnews.com/news/prevalent-brain-disease-identified-better-late-than-never/> [accessed 3 May 2019].

[367] 'Introducing LATE—A Common TDP-43 Proteinopathy That Strikes After 80 | ALZFORUM' <https://www.alzforum.org/news/research-news/introducing-late-common-tdp-43-proteinopathy-strikes-after-80> [accessed 6 May 2019].

[368] 'Bart De Strooper Lab' <http://www.vib.be/en/research/scientists/Pages/Bart-De-Strooper-Lab.aspx> [accessed 6 May 2019].

[369] 'Expert Reaction to a Study Describing a Recently Recognized Alzheimer's-like Brain Disorder | Science Media Centre' <https://www.sciencemediacentre.org/expert-reaction-to-a-study-describing-a-recently-recognized-alzheimers-like-brain-disorder/> [accessed 5 May 2019].

[370] 'Researchers Define Alzheimer's-like Brain Disorder: LATE Symptoms Resembles Alzheimer's Disease but Has Different Cause', *ScienceDaily* <https://www.sciencedaily.com/releases/2019/04/190430121800.htm> [accessed 3 May 2019].

[371] 'Researchers Just Found a New Type of Dementia' <http://www.advisory.com/daily-briefing/2019/05/06/alzheimers> [accessed 6 May 2019].

[372] 'When Is "Alzheimer's" Not Alzheimer's? Researchers Characterize a Different Form of Dementia', *ScienceDaily* <https://www.sciencedaily.com/releases/2019/04/190430173210.htm> [accessed 6 May 2019].

[373] 'LATE Dementia Is a New Type of Brain Disease That Mimics Alzheimer's', *Being Patient*, 2019 <https://www.beingpatient.com/late-dementia/> [accessed 6 May 2019].

[374] 'Posterior Cortical Atrophy', *Memory and Aging Center* <https://memory.ucsf.edu/dementia/posterior-cortical-atrophy> [accessed 13 November 2019].

[375] 'Posterior Cortical Atrophy', *Memory and Aging Center* <https://memory.ucsf.edu/dementia/posterior-cortical-atrophy> [accessed 13 November 2019].

[376] 'Posterior Cortical Atrophy', *Memory and Aging Center* <https://memory.ucsf.edu/dementia/posterior-cortical-atrophy> [accessed 26 July 2019].

[377] INSERM US14-- ALL RIGHTS RESERVED, 'Orphanet: Posterior Cortical Atrophy' <https://www.orpha.net/consor/cgi-bin/OC_Exp.php?Lng=GB&Expert=54247> [accessed 28 July 2019].

[378] 'Posterior Cortical Atrophy', *Alzheimer's Society* <https://www.alzheimers.org.uk/about-dementia/types-dementia/Posterior-cortical-atrophy> [accessed 26 July 2019].

[379] 'Posterior Cortical Atrophy'.

[380] Sebastian J. Crutch and others, 'Consensus Classification of Posterior Cortical Atrophy', *Alzheimer's & Dementia*, 13.8 (2017), 870–84 <https://doi.org/10.1016/j.jalz.2017.01.014>.

[381] 'Amyotrophic Lateral Sclerosis (ALS) Fact Sheet | National Institute of Neurological Disorders and Stroke' <https://www.ninds.nih.gov/Disorders/Patient-Caregiver-Education/Fact-Sheets/Amyotrophic-Lateral-Sclerosis-ALS-Fact-Sheet> [accessed 3 December 2019].

[382] Philip Van Damme Bosch Wim Robberecht, and Ludo Van Den, *English: This Figure Is from the Journal Article 'Modelling Amyotrophic Lateral Sclerosis: Progress and Possibilities' and Shows Ten Proposed Disease Mechanisms for ALS.*, 2017, http://dmm.biologists.org/content/10/5/537 Philip Van Damme P, Robberecht W, Van Den Bosch L (May 2017). 'Modelling amyotrophic lateral sclerosis: progress and possibilities.' Disease Models and Mechanisms. 10 (5): 537-549. doi:10.1242/dmm.029058 PMC: 5451175 PMID: 28468939. <https://commons.wikimedia.org/wiki/File:ALS_Disease_Pathology_and_Proposed_Disease_Mechanisms.jpg> [accessed 6 January 2020].

[383] 'Amyotrophic Lateral Sclerosis (ALS) - Causes/Inheritance', *Muscular Dystrophy Association*, 2015 <https://www.mda.org/disease/amyotrophic-lateral-sclerosis/causes-inheritance> [accessed 6 January 2020].

[384] 'How Common Is ALS?', *ALS News Today* <https://alsnewstoday.com/how-common-is-als/> [accessed 3 December 2019].

[385] Raygene Martier, Jolanda M. Liefhebber, Jana Miniarikova, and others, 'Artificial MicroRNAs Targeting C9orf72 Can Reduce Accumulation of Intra-Nuclear Transcripts in ALS and FTD Patients', *Molecular Therapy - Nucleic Acids*, 14 (2019), 593–608 <https://doi.org/10.1016/j.omtn.2019.01.010>.

[386] Raygene Martier, Jolanda M. Liefhebber, Ana García-Osta, and others, 'Targeting RNA-Mediated Toxicity in C9orf72 ALS and/or FTD by RNAi-Based Gene Therapy', *Molecular Therapy - Nucleic Acids*, 16 (2019), 26–37 <https://doi.org/10.1016/j.omtn.2019.02.001>.

[387] 'SOD1 - Superoxide Dismutase [Cu-Zn] - Homo Sapiens (Human) - SOD1 Gene & Protein' <https://www.uniprot.org/uniprot/P00441> [accessed 3 December 2019].

[388] 'What Is the Prevalence of Amyotrophic Lateral Sclerosis (ALS) (Lou Gehrig Disease)?' <https://www.medscape.com/answers/2111360-182652/what-is-the-prevalence-of-amyotrophic-lateral-sclerosis-als-lou-gehrig-disease> [accessed 3 December 2019].

[389] 'The ALS Association' <http://www.alsa.org/about-als/facts-you-should-know.html> [accessed 3 December 2019].

[390] 'ALS Incidence and Prevalence Worldwide', *Alstreatment.Com* <https://alstreatment.com/amyotrophic-lateral-sclerosis-incidence/> [accessed 3 December 2019].

[391] 'Pathology of Motor Neuron Disorders: Definition, Epidemiology, Etiology', 2019 <https://emedicine.medscape.com/article/2111360-overview#a2> [accessed 3 December 2019].

[392] 'ALS Incidence and Prevalence Worldwide'.

[393] 'Who Gets ALS?', *ALSA.Org* <http://webga.alsa.org/site/PageServer/?pagename=GA_1_WhoGets.html> [accessed 3 December 2019].

[394] 'Symptoms' <https://stanfordhealthcare.org/medical-conditions/brain-and-nerves/amyotrophic-lateral-sclerosis/symptoms.html> [accessed 6 December 2019].

[395] 'Amyotrophic Lateral Sclerosis', *NORD (National Organization for Rare Disorders)* <https://rarediseases.org/rare-diseases/amyotrophic-lateral-sclerosis/> [accessed 6 December 2019].

[396] 'Amyotrophic Lateral Sclerosis (ALS) - Symptoms and Causes', *Mayo Clinic* <https://www.mayoclinic.org/diseases-conditions/amyotrophic-lateral-sclerosis/symptoms-causes/syc-20354022> [accessed 6 December 2019].

[397] Lokesh C. Wijesekera and P. Nigel Leigh, 'Amyotrophic Lateral Sclerosis', *Orphanet Journal of Rare Diseases*, 4.1 (2009), 3 <https://doi.org/10.1186/1750-1172-4-3>.

[398] 'Early Symptoms of ALS/MND | ALS Worldwide' <https://alsworldwide.org/care-and-support/article/early-symptoms-of-als-mnd> [accessed 6 December 2019].

[399] Harvard Health Publishing, 'Amyotrophic Lateral Sclerosis (ALS)', *Harvard Health* <https://www.health.harvard.edu/a_to_z/amyotrophic-lateral-sclerosis-als-a-to-z> [accessed 6 December 2019].

[400] 'Report to Congress: Traumatic Brain Injury in the United States | Concussion | Traumatic Brain Injury | CDC Injury Center', 2019 <https://www.cdc.gov/traumaticbraininjury/pubs/tbi_report_to_congress.html> [accessed 10 December 2020].

[401] Michael Dewan and others, 'Estimating the Global Incidence of Traumatic Brain Injury', *Journal of Neurosurgery*, 130 (2018), 1–18 <https://doi.org/10.3171/2017.10.JNS17352>.

[402] J. A. Corsellis and J. B. Brierley, 'Observations on the Pathology of Insidious Dementia Following Head Injury', *The Journal of Mental Science*, 105 (1959), 714–20 <https://doi.org/10.1192/bjp.105.440.714>.

[403] J. a. N. Corsellis, C. J. Bruton, and Dorothy Freeman-Browne, 'The Aftermath

of Boxing1', *Psychological Medicine*, 3.3 (1973), 270–303 <https://doi.org/10.1017/S0033291700049588>.

[404] 'Chronic Traumatic Encephalopathy - Symptoms and Causes', *Mayo Clinic* <https://www.mayoclinic.org/diseases-conditions/chronic-traumatic-encephalopathy/symptoms-causes/syc-20370921> [accessed 10 December 2020].

[405] Bennet I. Omalu, Steven T. DeKosky, and others, 'Chronic Traumatic Encephalopathy in a National Football League Player', *Neurosurgery*, 57.1 (2005), 128–34; discussion 128-134 <https://doi.org/10.1227/01.neu.0000163407.92769.ed>.

[406] Robert A. Stern and others, 'Clinical Presentation of Chronic Traumatic Encephalopathy', *Neurology*, 81.13 (2013), 1122–29 <https://doi.org/10.1212/WNL.0b013e3182a55f7f>.

[407] Kevin F. Bieniek and others, 'Association between Contact Sports Participation and Chronic Traumatic Encephalopathy: A Retrospective Cohort Study', *Brain Pathology*, 30.1 (2020), 63–74 <https://doi.org/10.1111/bpa.12757>.

[408] 'CTE Prevalence High...and Not Just in Athletes', *Medscape* <http://www.medscape.com/viewarticle/915218> [accessed 10 December 2020].

[409] Bennet I. Omalu, Julian Bailes, and others, 'Chronic Traumatic Encephalopathy, Suicides and Parasuicides in Professional American Athletes: The Role of the Forensic Pathologist', *The American Journal of Forensic Medicine and Pathology*, 31.2 (2010), 130–32 <https://doi.org/10.1097/PAF.0b013e3181ca7f35>.

[410] Joseph C. Maroon and others, 'Chronic Traumatic Encephalopathy in Contact Sports: A Systematic Review of All Reported Pathological Cases', *PloS One*, 10.2 (2015), e0117338 <https://doi.org/10.1371/journal.pone.0117338>.

[411] H. Ling and others, 'Does Corticobasal Degeneration Exist? A Clinicopathological Re-Evaluation', *Brain*, 133.7 (2010), 2045–57 <https://doi.org/10.1093/brain/awq123>.

[412] W. R. Gibb, P. J. Luthert, and C. D. Marsden, 'Corticobasal Degeneration', *Brain: A Journal of Neurology*, 112 (Pt 5) (1989), 1171–92 <https://doi.org/10.1093/brain/112.5.1171>.

[413] 'Corticobasal Syndrome (CBS)', *Baylor College of Medicine* <https://www.bcm.edu/healthcare/care-centers/parkinsons/conditions/corticobasal-syndrome> [accessed 4 December 2019].

[414] Andreea L. Seritan and others, 'Functional Imaging as a Window to Dementia: Corticobasal Degeneration', *The Journal of Neuropsychiatry and Clinical Neurosciences*, 16.4 (2004), 393–99 <https://doi.org/10.1176/jnp.16.4.393>.

[415] 'Corticobasal Degeneration', *NORD (National Organization for Rare Disorders)* <https://rarediseases.org/rare-diseases/corticobasal-degeneration/> [accessed 6 December 2019].

[416] 'Corticobasal Syndrome', *Memory and Aging Center*

<https://memory.ucsf.edu/dementia/corticobasal-syndrome> [accessed 4 December 2019].

[417] Alexander Pantelyat and others, 'Acalculia in Autopsy-Proven Corticobasal Degeneration', *Neurology*, 76.7 0 2 (2011), S61–63 <https://doi.org/10.1212/WNL.0b013e31820c34ca>.

[418] 'What Is Parkinson's & What Does It Do' <https://www.parkinsonswa.org.au/what-is-parkinsons/> [accessed 6 December 2019].

[419] Jonathan Graff-Radford and others, 'The Alien Limb Phenomenon', *Journal of Neurology*, 260.7 (2013), 1880–88 <https://doi.org/10.1007/s00415-013-6898-y>.

[420] 'Apraxia', *NORD (National Organization for Rare Disorders)* <https://rarediseases.org/rare-diseases/apraxia/> [accessed 6 December 2019].

[421] 'Limb Apraxia', *American Speech-Language-Hearing Association* <https://www.asha.org/Glossary/Limb-Apraxia/> [accessed 6 December 2019].

[422] A. Berardelli and others, 'Pathophysiology of Bradykinesia in Parkinson's Disease', *Brain*, 124.11 (2001), 2131–46 <https://doi.org/10.1093/brain/124.11.2131>.

[423] European Parkinson's Disease Association, 'Bradykinesia' <https://www.epda.eu.com/about-parkinsons/symptoms/motor-symptoms/bradykinesia/> [accessed 6 December 2019].

[424] 'What Is Dystonia? | Dystonia Medical Research Foundation' <https://dystonia-foundation.org/what-is-dystonia/> [accessed 6 December 2019].

[425] 'Dystonia – Classifications, Symptoms and Treatment' <https://www.aans.org/> [accessed 6 December 2019].

[426] Theodore P. Parthimos and Kleopatra H. Schulpis, 'The Significant Characteristics of Corticobasal Syndrome', *Annals of Research Hospitals*, 3.0 (2019) <http://arh.amegroups.com/article/view/4676> [accessed 6 December 2019].

[427] 'Creutzfeldt-Jakob Disease Fact Sheet | National Institute of Neurological Disorders and Stroke' <https://www.ninds.nih.gov/Disorders/Patient-Caregiver-Education/Fact-Sheets/Creutzfeldt-Jakob-Disease-Fact-Sheet> [accessed 24 February 2018].

[428] 'Brain Cell Advance Brings Fresh Hope for Creutzfeldt-Jakob Disease Therapies: Experts Have Developed a Way of Studying the Disease in the Lab Using Brain Cells Derived from Human Stem Cells', *ScienceDaily* <https://www.sciencedaily.com/releases/2017/11/171120111306.htm> [accessed 24 February 2018].

[429] 'Creutzfeldt-Jakob Disease, Classic (CJD) | Prion Diseases | CDC' <https://www.cdc.gov/prions/cjd/> [accessed 24 February 2018].

[430] 'Creutzfeldt-Jakob Disease Information Page | National Institute of Neurological Disorders and Stroke' <https://www.ninds.nih.gov/Disorders/All-Disorders/Creutzfeldt-Jakob-Disease-Information-Page> [accessed 24 February 2018].

[431] 'Diagnosing Sporadic Creutzfeldt-Jakob Disease'

<https://www.aan.com/Guidelines/Home/GetGuidelineContent/567> [accessed 6 January 2020].

[432] 'Prion Diseases', *Memory and Aging Center* <https://memory.ucsf.edu/dementia/rapidly-progressive-dementias/prion-diseases> [accessed 6 January 2020].

[433] 'File:Prion Protein Immunostaining (Purple) and Spongiform Change in the Brain of a Patient with Creutzfeldt-Jakob Disease.Jpg', *Wikipedia*, 2012 <https://en.wikipedia.org/w/index.php?title=File:Prion_protein_immunostaining_(purple)_and_spongiform_change_in_the_brain_of_a_patient_with_Creutzfeldt-Jakob_Disease.jpg&oldid=475155045> [accessed 5 January 2020].

[434] 'Era of Iatrogenic CJD Transmission "Nearly Closed"', *Medscape* <http://www.medscape.com/viewarticle/764462> [accessed 6 January 2020].

[435] 'About VCJD | Variant Creutzfeldt-Jakob Disease, Classic (CJD) | Prion Disease | CDC', 2019 <https://www.cdc.gov/prions/vcjd/about.html> [accessed 5 January 2020].

[436] Content Providers, *ID#:   10130*, 2004, Public Health Image Library (PHIL) ID#: 10131 <https://commons.wikimedia.org/wiki/File:Variant_Creutzfeldt-Jakob_disease_(vCJD),_typical_amyloid_plaques,_H%26E.jpg> [accessed 5 January 2020].

[437] 'Creutzfeldt-Jakob Disease', *Nhs.Uk*, 2017 <https://www.nhs.uk/conditions/creutzfeldt-jakob-disease-cjd/> [accessed 5 January 2020].

[438] 'Mad Cow Disease (Bovine Spongiform Encephalopathy) - Health Encyclopedia - University of Rochester Medical Center' <https://www.urmc.rochester.edu/encyclopedia/content.aspx?ContentTypeID=85&ContentID=P01444> [accessed 5 January 2020].

[439] 'Genetics Basics Lesson 3: Modes of Inheritance' <http://hihg.med.miami.edu/code/http/modules/education/Design/Print.asp?CourseNum=1&LessonNum=3> [accessed 18 March 2019].

[440] Genetics Home Reference, 'Huntington Disease', *Genetics Home Reference* <https://ghr.nlm.nih.gov/condition/huntington-disease> [accessed 12 January 2019].

[441] 'Akinetic–Rigid Syndromes - Oxford Medicine' <http://oxfordmedicine.com/view/10.1093/med/9780192619112.001.0001/med-9780192619112-section-003> [accessed 30 January 2019].

[442] 'Trinucleotide Repeat Disorders', *HOPES Huntington's Disease Information*, 2010 <http://web.stanford.edu/group/hopes/cgi-bin/hopes_test/trinucleotide-repeat-disorders/> [accessed 30 January 2019].

[443] 'UPMC - Department of Pathology - University of Pittsburgh' <https://path.upmc.edu/index.html> [accessed 19 March 2019].

[444] 'Huntington's Disease', *Alzheimer's Disease and Dementia* <https://alz.org/alzheimers-dementia/what-is-dementia/types-of-dementia/huntington-s-disease> [accessed 12 January 2019].

[445] 'Juvenile Huntington Disease | Genetic and Rare Diseases Information Center (GARD) – an NCATS Program' <https://rarediseases.info.nih.gov/diseases/10510/juvenile-huntington-disease> [accessed 19 March 2019].

[446] 'Juvenile Onset HD |' <https://hdsa.org/living-with-hd/juvenile-onset-hd/> [accessed 19 March 2019].

[447] 'What Is HD? |' <https://hdsa.org/what-is-hd/> [accessed 12 January 2019].

[448] 'Population Genetics and Huntington's Disease', *HOPES Huntington's Disease Information*, 2010 <http://web.stanford.edu/group/hopes/cgi-bin/hopes_test/population-genetics-and-hd/> [accessed 12 January 2019].

[449] Victoria Divino and others, 'The Direct Medical Costs of Huntington's Disease by Stage. A Retrospective Commercial and Medicaid Claims Data Analysis', *Journal of Medical Economics*, 16.8 (2013), 1043–50 <https://doi.org/10.3111/13696998.2013.818545>.

[450] 'Early Warning Signs Of Huntington's Disease: Metabolic Changes Ahead Of Symptoms May Lead Scientists To Treatment', *Medical Daily*, 2017 <http://www.medicaldaily.com/early-warning-signs-huntingtons-disease-metabolic-changes-ahead-symptoms-may-412404> [accessed 24 February 2018].

[451] 'Huntington's Disease | Memory and Aging Center' <https://memory.ucsf.edu/huntington-disease> [accessed 24 February 2018].

[452] 'Symptoms of HD | Huntington's Disease Association' <https://www.hda.org.uk/huntingtons-disease/what-is-huntingtons-disease/symptoms-of-huntingtons-disease> [accessed 24 February 2018].

[453] 'Huntington's Disease', *Nhs.Uk* <https://www.nhs.uk/conditions/huntingdons-disease/> [accessed 24 February 2018].

[454] 'Understanding Huntington's Disease', *HealthPrep* <https://healthprep.com/conditions/understanding-huntingtons-disease/> [accessed 25 February 2018].

[455] 'What Is Huntington Disease? Symptoms, Signs, Causes & Treatment', *EMedicineHealth* <https://www.emedicinehealth.com/dementia_overview/article_em.htm> [accessed 24 February 2018].

[456] Shiraz Tyebji and Anthony J. Hannan, 'Synaptopathic Mechanisms of Neurodegeneration and Dementia: Insights from Huntington's Disease', *Progress in Neurobiology*, 153 (2017), 18–45 <https://doi.org/10.1016/j.pneurobio.2017.03.008>.

[457] 'Dementia Due to Huntington Disease', *DoveMed* <http://www.dovemed.com/diseases-conditions/dementia-due-to-huntington-disease-hd/> [accessed 24 February 2018].

[458] 'Huntington's Disease - Symptoms and Causes', *Mayo Clinic* <http://www.mayoclinic.org/diseases-conditions/huntingtons-disease/symptoms-causes/syc-20356117> [accessed 24 February 2018].

[459] 'Huntington's Disease: Symptoms, Causes, and Treatment', *Medical News Today* <https://www.medicalnewstoday.com/articles/159552.php> [accessed 24 February 2018].

[460] 'Huntington's Disease', *Your.MD* <https://www.your.md/condition/huntingtons-disease/> [accessed 25 February 2018].

[461] '6 Early Warning Signs of Huntington's Disease' <http://www.activebeat.com/your-health/6-early-warning-signs-of-huntingtons-disease/> [accessed 24 February 2018].

[462] 'Huntington's Disease: Symptoms, Stages & 5 Natural Treatments', *David Avocado Wolfe*, 2017 <https://www.davidwolfe.com/huntingtons-disease/> [accessed 25 February 2018].

[463] Erika Driver-Dunckley and John N. Caviness, 'CHAPTER 67 - HUNTINGTON'S DISEASE', in *Neurology and Clinical Neuroscience*, ed. by Anthony H. V. Schapira and others (Philadelphia: Mosby, 2007), pp. 879–85 <https://doi.org/10.1016/B978-0-323-03354-1.50071-7>.

[464] Celia Stewart, 'Dysphagia Symptoms and Treatment in Huntington's Disease: Review', *SIG 13 Perspectives on Swallowing and Swallowing Disorders (Dysphagia)*, 21.4 (2012), 126–34 <https://doi.org/10.1044/sasd21.4.126>.

[465] 'Huntington's Disease: Symptoms, Treatment', *WebMD* <https://www.webmd.com/brain/hungtingtons-disease-causes-symptoms-treatment> [accessed 24 February 2018].

[466] 'Psychiatric Disorders Raise Risk of Suicidal Behavior in HD Trial Patients', *Huntington's Disease News*, 2019 <https://huntingtonsdiseasenews.com/2019/03/28/active-psychiatric-disorders-increase-risk-of-suicidal-behaviors-in-hd-trial-patients/> [accessed 4 January 2020].

[467] 'Suicide Prevention | Huntington's Disease Society of America' <https://hdsa.org/find-help/clinical-care-services/suicide-prevention/> [accessed 4 January 2020].

[468] Jarem Sawatsky, *Dancing with Elephants: Mindfulness Training For Those Living With Dementia, Chronic Illness or an Aging Brain* (Red Canoe Press, 2017).

[469] 'Hydro- | Definition of Hydro- in English by Oxford Dictionaries', *Oxford Dictionaries | English* <https://en.oxforddictionaries.com/definition/hydro-> [accessed 9 May 2019].

[470] '-Cephalus', *TheFreeDictionary.Com* <https://medical-dictionary.thefreedictionary.com/-cephalus> [accessed 9 May 2019].

[471] 'Hydrocephalus – Causes, Symptom and Surgical Treatments' <https://www.aans.org/> [accessed 23 November 2019].

[472] 'What Is Communicating Hydrocephalus?' <https://www.medscape.com/answers/1135286-82879/what-is-communicating-hydrocephalus> [accessed 23 November 2019].

[473] 'Hydrocephalus | Genetic and Rare Diseases Information Center (GARD) – an NCATS Program' <https://rarediseases.info.nih.gov/diseases/6682/hydrocephalus> [accessed 18 February 2018].

[474] 'Hydrocephalus' <https://www.hopkinsmedicine.org/health/conditions-and-diseases/hydrocephalus> [accessed 23 November 2019].

[475] 'Normal Pressure Hydrocephalus | Hydrocephalus Association' <https://www.hydroassoc.org/normal-pressure-hydrocephalus/> [accessed 18 February 2018].

[476] 'Normal Pressure Hydrocephalus (NPH)', *Cleveland Clinic* <https://my.clevelandclinic.org/health/diseases/15849-normal-pressure-hydrocephalus-nph> [accessed 10 May 2019].

[477] 'Normal Pressure Hydrocephalus (NPH)', *Cleveland Clinic* <https://my.clevelandclinic.org/health/diseases/15849-normal-pressure-hydrocephalus-nph> [accessed 9 May 2019].

[478] 'Hydrocephalus Fact Sheet | National Institute of Neurological Disorders and Stroke' <https://www.ninds.nih.gov/Disorders/Patient-Caregiver-Education/Fact-Sheets/Hydrocephalus-Fact-Sheet> [accessed 9 May 2019].

[479] Caren McHenry Martin, 'The "Reversible" Dementia of Idiopathic Normal Pressure Hydrocephalus', *The Consultant Pharmacist: The Journal of the American Society of Consultant Pharmacists*, 21.11 (2006), 888–92, 901–3.

[480] 'Facts and Stats', *Hydrocephalus Association* <https://www.hydroassoc.org/about-us/newsroom/facts-and-stats-2/> [accessed 10 May 2019].

[481] 'Causes', *Hydrocephalus Association* <https://www.hydroassoc.org/causes/> [accessed 10 May 2019].

[482] 'Normal Pressure Hydrocephalus (NPH) | AdventHealth Neuroscience Institute' <http://www.adventhealthneuroinstitute.com/programs/normal-pressure-hydrocephalus> [accessed 10 May 2019].

[483] Hiroaki Kazui, '[Cognitive impairment in patients with idiopathic normal pressure hydrocephalus]', *Brain and Nerve = Shinkei Kenkyu No Shinpo*, 60.3 (2008), 225–31.

[484] A. Berardelli and others, 'Pathophysiology of Bradykinesia in Parkinson's Disease', *Brain: A Journal of Neurology*, 124.Pt 11 (2001), 2131–46.

[485] 'Cognitive Therapy for NPH Patients | Hydrocephalus Association' <https://www.hydroassoc.org/cognitive-therapy-for-nph-patients/> [accessed 18 February 2018].

[486] 'AANS | Adult-Onset Hydrocephalus' <http://www.aans.org/Patients/Neurosurgical-Conditions-and-Treatments/Adult-Onset-Hydrocephalus> [accessed 18 February 2018].

[487] 'Hydrocephalus > Condition at Yale Medicine', *Yale Medicine* <https://www.yalemedicine.org/conditions/hydrocephalus/> [accessed 18 February 2018].

[488] 'Normal Pressure Hydrocephalus: Practice Essentials, Background, Pathophysiology', 2019 <https://emedicine.medscape.com/article/1150924-overview> [accessed 10 May 2019].

[489] 'Symptoms and Diagnosis | Hydrocephalus Association' <https://www.hydroassoc.org/symptoms-and-diagnosis-nph/> [accessed 18 February 2018].

[490] 'Normal Pressure Hydrocephalus - an Overview | ScienceDirect Topics' <https://www.sciencedirect.com/topics/neuroscience/normal-pressure-hydrocephalus> [accessed 18 February 2018].

[491] 'Normal Pressure Hydrocephalus in Adults | GPonline' <https://www.gponline.com/normal-pressure-hydrocephalus-adults/article/586761> [accessed 26 December 2019].

[492] 'SHYMA.Pdf' <http://www.hydroassoc.org/docs/SHYMA.pdf> [accessed 18 February 2018].

[493] 'Hydrocephalus – Causes, Symptom and Surgical Treatments' <https://www.aans.org/> [accessed 10 May 2019].

[494] 'Hydrocephalus (for Parents) - KidsHealth' <https://kidshealth.org/en/parents/hydrocephalus.html> [accessed 10 May 2019].

[495] 'Normal Pressure Hydrocephalus', *Child Neurology Foundation* <https://www.childneurologyfoundation.org/disorder/normal-pressure-hydrocephalus/> [accessed 10 May 2019].

[496] Harvard Health Publishing, 'Hydrocephalus', *Harvard Health* <https://www.health.harvard.edu/a_to_z/hydrocephalus-a-to-z> [accessed 10 May 2019].

[497] 'Hydrocephalus', *NORD (National Organization for Rare Disorders)* <https://rarediseases.org/rare-diseases/hydrocephalus/> [accessed 10 May 2019].

[498] 'Normal Pressure Hydrocephalus', *Johns Hopkins Medicine Health Library* <https://www.hopkinsmedicine.org/health/conditions-and-diseases/hydrocephalus/normal-pressure-hydrocephalus> [accessed 10 May 2019].

[499] 'Hydrocephalus'.

[500] 'Wernicke-Korsakoff Syndrome Information Page | National Institute of Neurological Disorders and Stroke' <https://www.ninds.nih.gov/Disorders/All-Disorders/Wernicke-Korsakoff-Syndrome-Information-Page> [accessed 24 February 2018].

[501] 'How Common Is Wernicke-Korsakoff Syndrome?', *Alcohol.Org* <https://www.alcohol.org/effects/wernicke-korsakoff-syndrome/> [accessed 11 May 2019].

[502] Sarayu Vasan and Anil Kumar, 'Wernicke Encephalopathy', in *StatPearls* (Treasure Island (FL): StatPearls Publishing, 2019) <http://www.ncbi.nlm.nih.gov/books/NBK470344/> [accessed 12 May 2019].

[503] 'Wernicke-Korsakoff Syndrome', *NORD (National Organization for Rare Disorders)* <https://rarediseases.org/rare-diseases/wernicke-korsakoff-syndrome/>

[accessed 12 May 2019].

[504] 'Korsakoff Syndrome', *Alzheimer's Disease and Dementia* <https://alz.org/alzheimers-dementia/what-is-dementia/types-of-dementia/korsakoff-syndrome> [accessed 12 May 2019].

[505] 'Korsakoff Syndrome'.

[506] 'Office of Dietary Supplements - Thiamin' <https://ods.od.nih.gov/factsheets/Thiamin-HealthProfessional/> [accessed 12 May 2019].

[507] Smit Patel, Karan Topiwala, and Lawrence Hudson, 'Wernicke's Encephalopathy', *Cureus*, 10.8 <https://doi.org/10.7759/cureus.3187>.

[508] Nicolaas JM Arts, Serge JW Walvoort, and Roy PC Kessels, 'Korsakoff's Syndrome: A Critical Review', *Neuropsychiatric Disease and Treatment*, 13 (2017), 2875–90 <https://doi.org/10.2147/NDT.S130078>.

[509] 'How Common Is Wernicke-Korsakoff Syndrome?', *Alcohol.Org* <https://www.alcohol.org/effects/wernicke-korsakoff-syndrome/> [accessed 11 May 2019].

[510] Shweta Akhouri and Edward J. Newton, 'Wernicke-Korsakoff Syndrome', in *StatPearls* (Treasure Island (FL): StatPearls Publishing, 2019) <http://www.ncbi.nlm.nih.gov/books/NBK430729/> [accessed 11 May 2019].

[511] Scot Thomas and M.D., 'Wet Brain from Alcohol: Signs, Symptoms, and Recovery', *American Addiction Centers* <https://americanaddictioncenters.org/alcoholism-treatment/wet-brain> [accessed 11 May 2019].

[512] 'Gayet –Wernicke Encephalopathy in Non Alcoholic Patients: A Serious Complication' <http://www.rarediseasesjournal.com/articles/gayet-wernicke-encephalopathy-in-non-alcoholic-patients-a-serious-complication-rarediseases-1-1037.php> [accessed 11 May 2019].

[513] 'Rarer_dementias_wernicke_korsakoff_e.Pdf' <https://alzheimer.ca/sites/default/files/files/national/other-dementias/rarer_dementias_wernicke_korsakoff_e.pdf> [accessed 11 May 2019].

[514] 'Neurology Center - Penn State Hershey Medical Center - Wernicke-Korsakoff Syndrome - Penn State Hershey Medical Center' <http://pennstatehershey.adam.com/content.aspx?productId=116&pid=1&gid=000771> [accessed 11 May 2019].

[515] 'Wernicke Korsakoff Syndrome - an Overview | ScienceDirect Topics' <https://www.sciencedirect.com/topics/neuroscience/wernicke-korsakoff-syndrome> [accessed 11 May 2019].

[516] 'Wernicke-Korsakoff Syndrome', *UF Health, University of Florida Health*, 2012 <https://ufhealth.org/wernicke-korsakoff-syndrome> [accessed 11 May 2019].

[517] 'Wernicke-Korsakoff Syndrome Information | Mount Sinai - New York', *Mount Sinai Health System* <https://www.mountsinai.org/health-library/diseases-conditions/wernicke-korsakoff-syndrome> [accessed 11 May 2019].

[518] Tatsuo Shimomura and others, 'Development of Wernicke-Korsakoff Syndrome

After Long Intervals Following Gastrectomy', *Archives of Neurology*, 55.9 (1998), 1242–45 <https://doi.org/10.1001/pubs.Arch Neurol.-ISSN-0003-9942-55-9-nob7478>.

[519] Mikael Häggström, *English: Most Significant Possible Long-Term Effects of Ethanol. Sources Are Found in Main Article: Wikipedia:Ethanol#Long-Term. Model: Mikael Häggström. To Discuss Image, Please See Template_talk:Häggström Diagrams*, 2009, All used images are in public domain. <https://commons.wikimedia.org/wiki/File:Possible_long-term_effects_of_ethanol.svg> [accessed 5 January 2020].

[520] 'Wernicke-Korsakoff Syndrome: Background, Etiology, Pathophysiology', 2019 <https://emedicine.medscape.com/article/288379-overview> [accessed 11 May 2019].

[521] 'Korsakoff Syndrome | Signs, Symptoms, & Diagnosis', *Dementia* <//www.alz.org/dementia/wernicke-korsakoff-syndrome-symptoms.asp> [accessed 24 February 2018].

[522] 'Wernicke-Korsakoff Syndrome - NORD (National Organization for Rare Disorders)', *NORD (National Organization for Rare Disorders)* <https://rarediseases.org/rare-diseases/wernicke-korsakoff-syndrome/> [accessed 24 February 2018].

[523] 'Wernicke-Korsakoff Syndrome | Genetic and Rare Diseases Information Center (GARD) – an NCATS Program' <https://rarediseases.info.nih.gov/diseases/6843/wernicke-korsakoff-syndrome> [accessed 24 February 2018].

[524] 'What Is Wernicke-Korsakoff Syndrome?', *WebMD* <https://www.webmd.com/brain/wernicke-korsakoff-syndrome-facts> [accessed 24 February 2018].

[525] 'What Is Wernicke-Korsakoff Syndrome?', *Medical News Today* <https://www.medicalnewstoday.com/articles/220007.php> [accessed 24 February 2018].

[526] William G. Gossman and Edward J. Newton, 'Wernicke-Korsakoff Syndrome', in *StatPearls* (Treasure Island (FL): StatPearls Publishing, 2017) <http://www.ncbi.nlm.nih.gov/books/NBK430729/> [accessed 24 February 2018].

[527] Alexander Donnelly, 'Wernicke-Korsakoff Syndrome: Recognition and Treatment', *Nursing Standard (Royal College of Nursing (Great Britain): 1987)*, 31.31 (2017), 46–53 <https://doi.org/10.7748/ns.2017.e10440>.

[528] Claudia Chaves and MD, 'Alcohol Dementia: What Is Wernicke-Korsakoff Syndrome?', *Verywell Health* <https://www.verywell.com/what-is-wernicke-korsakoff-98769> [accessed 24 February 2018].

[529] 'Wernicke Encephalopathy and Korsakoff Syndrome – Knowledge for Medical Students and Physicians' <https://www.amboss.com/us/knowledge/Wernicke_encephalopathy_and_Korsakoff_syndrome> [accessed 24 February 2018].

[530] Michael Pekker, 'Wernicke-Korsakoff Syndrome (WKS) - Alzheimer's Disease: Causes, Symptoms, Treatment', *Wernicke-Korsakoff Syndrome (WKS) - Alzheimer's Disease*, 2017 <http://alzheimers-review.blogspot.com/2017/10/wernicke-korsakoff-

syndrome-wks.html> [accessed 24 February 2018].

[531] 'Decreased Proteins, Not Amyloid Plaques, Tied to Alzheimer's Disease', *ScienceDaily* <https://www.sciencedaily.com/releases/2022/10/221004151217.htm> [accessed 3 February 2023].

[532] Andrea Sturchio and others, 'High Soluble Amyloid-β 42 Predicts Normal Cognition in Amyloid-Positive Individuals with Alzheimer's Disease-Causing Mutations', *Journal of Alzheimer's Disease*, 90.1 (2022), 333–48 <https://doi.org/10.3233/JAD-220808>.

[533] 'Predicting the Future: A Quick, Easy Scan Can Reveal Late-Life Dementia Risk', *ScienceDaily* <https://www.sciencedaily.com/releases/2022/06/220626200205.htm> [accessed 27 January 2023].

[534] Tenielle Porter and others, 'Abdominal Aortic Calcification on Lateral Spine Images Captured during Bone Density Testing and Late-Life Dementia Risk in Older Women: A Prospective Cohort Study', *The Lancet Regional Health – Western Pacific*, 26 (2022) <https://doi.org/10.1016/j.lanwpc.2022.100502>.

[535] Fabienne Landry-McGill, 'Low Muscle Mass Linked to Cognitive Decline', *Futurity*, 2022 <https://www.futurity.org/muscle-mass-cognitive-decline-exercise-dementia-2770062/> [accessed 29 January 2023].

[536] Anne-Julie Tessier and others, 'Association of Low Muscle Mass With Cognitive Function During a 3-Year Follow-up Among Adults Aged 65 to 86 Years in the Canadian Longitudinal Study on Aging', *JAMA Network Open*, 5.7 (2022), e2219926 <https://doi.org/10.1001/jamanetworkopen.2022.19926>.

[537] 'Could a Computer Diagnose Alzheimer's Disease and Dementia?', *ScienceDaily* <https://www.sciencedaily.com/releases/2022/07/220711163210.htm> [accessed 28 January 2023].

[538] Samad Amini and others, 'Automated Detection of Mild Cognitive Impairment and Dementia from Voice Recordings: A Natural Language Processing Approach', *Alzheimer's & Dementia*, n/a.n/a <https://doi.org/10.1002/alz.12721>.

[539] Yifan Wang and others, 'Systematic Evaluation of Urinary Formic Acid as a New Potential Biomarker for Alzheimer's Disease', *Frontiers in Aging Neuroscience*, 14 (2022) <https://www.frontiersin.org/articles/10.3389/fnagi.2022.1046066> [accessed 6 February 2023].

[540] 'Alzheimer's or Lewy Body Dementia? How Patients Draw Can Determine the Type of Dementia | Research News', *University of Tsukuba* <https://www.tsukuba.ac.jp/en/research-news/20221101140000.html> [accessed 5 February 2023].

[541] Yasunori Yamada and others, 'Characteristics of Drawing Process Differentiate Alzheimer's Disease and Dementia with Lewy Bodies', *Journal of Alzheimer's Disease*, 90.2 (2022), 693–704 <https://doi.org/10.3233/JAD-220546>.

[542] 'Scientists Detect Dementia Signs as Early as Nine Years Ahead of Diagnosis', *University of Cambridge*, 2022 <https://www.cam.ac.uk/research/news/scientists-detect-dementia-signs-as-early-as-nine-years-ahead-of-diagnosis> [accessed 5 February 2023].

[543] Nol Swaddiwudhipong and others, 'Pre-Diagnostic Cognitive and Functional Impairment in Multiple Sporadic Neurodegenerative Diseases', *Alzheimer's & Dementia*, n/a.n/a <https://doi.org/10.1002/alz.12802>.

Printed in Great Britain
by Amazon